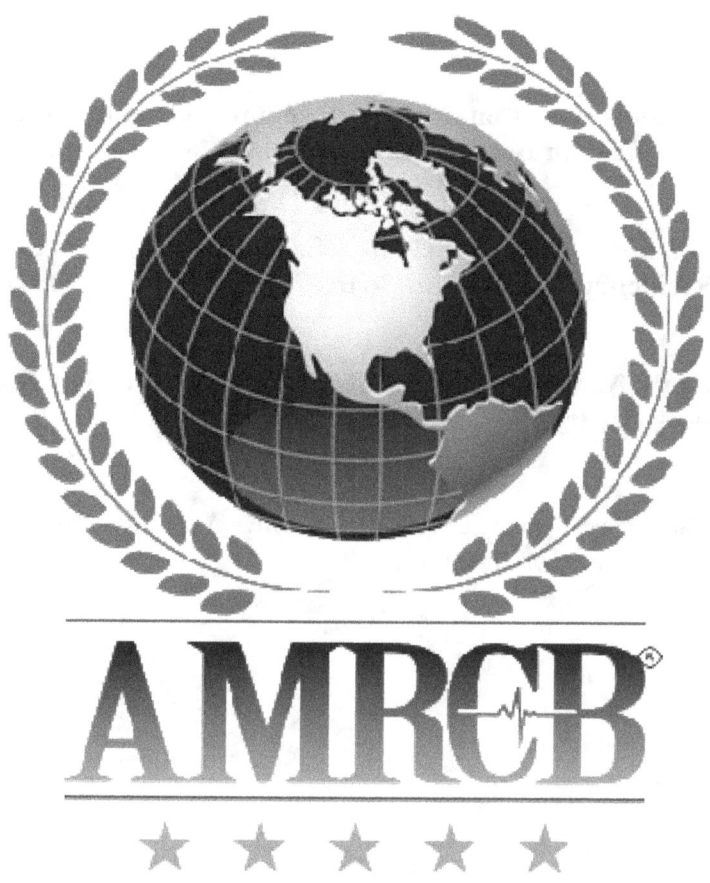

Suggested Citation
Canadian Medical Schools - American Medical Residency Certification Board®, 2015

ADDITIONAL AMRCB® PUBLICATIONS

Caribbean Medical Schools Based on a U.S. Curriculum – Greater and Lesser Antilles. American Medical Residency Certification Board®, 2014. ISBN-13: 978-1500419042, ISBN-10: 1500419044

Central and South American Medical Schools (Caribbean Region) based on a U.S. Curriculum - American Medical Residency Certification Board®, 2015. ISBN-13:978-1505589931, ISBN-10: 1505589932

AMRCB® Certification - American Medical Residency Certification Board®, 2015. ISBN-13: 978-1507624296, ISBN-10: 1507624298

Irish Medical Schools – Based on a U.S. Curriculum. American Medical Residency Certification Board®, 2015. Expected Publication in summer 2015

DEDICATION

This book is dedicated to potential medical school students across the globe. While the aim of this book is to describe Canadian Medical Schools, additional information is provided to assist in guiding students on choosing a potential medical residency in the United States and in Canada. We hope that potential students in Canada, the United States, and across the international community will find this reference a useful tool. The AMRCB® wishes all students success in their chosen fields.

ACKNOWLEDGMENTS

Steven W. Powell, MD, MPH, CPE, FAPA - Primary Author

Adnan Khan, MD

Dennis Sehgal, MD – Foreword

Amy Fecteau, AS – Editing and Creative Ideas

CONTENTS

FOREWORD

Dear Future Colleague,

Congratulations on deciding to pursue medicine as your future career choice. It takes a disciplined background and determined mindset to make such a decision. The Canadian health care system has all the right tools and resources to ensure that you become a talented and skillful physician. Located in North America, Canada has an advantage as it has access to the ever improving technology and education available in this system. Canada's multicultural population also provides additional benefits. Physicians have influenced the system from various countries around the world allowing Canada to become a global leader in healthcare.

Canadian medical schools are located in various cities across the country and follow standard guidelines and regulations. This means that regardless of the school, you can expect the finest education, training, and support. The guidance and aid is provided by professors, administrative and career staff along with your classmates who are focused on similar goals.

Living in Canada is also very pleasant. While it is true that winters in some parts of the country can get pretty rough, it does open up the opportunity to enjoy a wide range of winter activities. These include skiing, snowboarding, outdoor skating rinks, ice fishing, snowmobiling, and the list goes on. Banff, Alberta and Whistler, British Columbia are a couple of the many places where this type of recreation takes place. There are also many parts of the country that have some of the greatest summers. Whether you are in downtown Toronto in the CN tower or on the beach in Vancouver, there are many ways to enjoy a break. There is sightseeing, museums, agriculture and of course one of the wonders of the world in Niagara Falls. To top everything off the people are very welcoming and always willing to show you the way to what your desires are. Canada is fortunate to be one of the countries that enjoys all four seasons to their fullest potential. In addition to the liveliness, the multiculturalism also gives you the opportunity to try food from almost anywhere in the world.

Even though all of these activities are available, it is not going to be a breeze to get through medical school. However, it is good to have a bit of downtime and know that there are hobbies and pleasurable activities that meet everyone's interests. Your venture through school will require endless dedication and some sacrifice. To follow your passion and become a caregiver you are set up to hit roadblocks. Everyone's path will be different in some way. My only advice to you in this matter is to keep your head up and continue to combat through the struggles: this will allow you to reach your dream of caring for people. Remember again that resources are available to help you get through school and they have been designed after watching past graduates and gaining insights from current physicians. You will never be entirely on your own.

After speaking to multiple colleagues that have gone through the process at University of Ottawa and Toronto, I have been able to confirm that each step of the pathway is a foundation for the next. They all agree that the preparation for clerkships, residency and licensing exams is phenomenal. Personally, I was born and raised in Canada but attended medical school abroad. I have been working in Canada for the last few years and also did some elective clerkships at McMaster University and the University of Toronto. The experiences during the clerkships were amazing and these experiences were important in developing my current capabilities. I was able to witness and be a part of multiple hospitals and the health system within the area. Actually seeing the professionalism and well-built system in place was truly exhilarating. The health system was made up of many facilities that include state of the art research centers, educational institutes, clinics, rehab offices and of course the multi-specialty hospitals. This really gave me the ability to decide which pathway to choose for my career as the choices tend to be endless.

We at AMRCB® believe that Canadian medical schools will provide you with the educational basis, motivation, and training that are important for your future. You will be at the forefront of the newest technology, research updates, and other influences in healthcare that will allow you to practice medicine at an elite level. This will be admired by anyone that you cross paths with and allow you to achieve what you have worked so hard for. If you choose Canada as your pathway to success, make sure that you take advantage of the resources to excel through medical school, but also enjoy your down time as it is important to grow as an individual as you prosper and enter into your profession.

On your journey to becoming a physician, we would like to offer you our best wishes. I truly look forward to having you as an integral part of global healthcare...

Sincerely,

Dennis Sehgal, MD
Chief Medical Officer
National Medical Group Inc.

INTRODUCTION

The goal of this publication is to present accurate information about the application process, match statistics, the medical education, and the seventeen individual allopathic medical schools located in Canada. The most up-to-date information at the time of publication has been provided and is updated each year for accuracy.

The medical school descriptors that are used describe detailed information about each institution to allow for comparisons and to highlight individual institutional strengths. Contact information is provided as are interview and match statistics for each school. Additional detailed information can be found on the individual websites of each medical school.

It is ultimately up to each individual student to decide which medical schools that they will apply to. It is recommended that students discuss their plans with current and past medical students of the school they are considering if possible, either in person or by using online forums. Successful applicants have performed research on the schools and have prepared extensively for the interview process.

Canadian Medical Schools

Alberta

- University of Alberta, Faculty of Medicine and Dentistry
- University of Calgary, Cumming School of Medicine

British Columbia

- University of British Columbia, Faculty of Medicine

Manitoba

- University of Manitoba, Faculty of Medicine

Newfoundland

- Memorial University of Newfoundland, Faculty of Medicine

Nova Scotia

- Dalhousie University, Faculty of Medicine

Ontario

- McMaster University, Michael G. DeGroote School of Medicine
- Northern Ontario School of Medicine
- University of Ottawa, Faculty of Medicine
- Queen's University, School of Medicine
- University of Toronto, Faculty of Medicine
- Western University, Schulich School of Medicine and Dentistry

Quebec

- Université Laval, Faculté de médecine
- McGill University, Faculty of Medicine
- Université de Montréal, Faculté de médecine
- Université de Sherbrooke, Faculté de médecine

Saskatchewan

- University of Saskatchewan, College of Medicine

Chapter 1
CANADIAN MEDICAL EDUCATION

Over 11,500 students are enrolled in medical schools in Canada each year with approximately 2,800 new physicians graduating each year. That number has risen steadily from 1968 when only 4,681 students were enrolled each year. The majority of students accepted in Canadian medical schools are Canadian citizens. On average across the country, approximately 20 foreign students are accepted each year as are approximately 10 United States citizens. More accepted students come from Quebec and Ontario than from other provinces or territories in Canada. While only 20% of those accepted to Canadian medical schools were women in 1970, women constitute nearly 56% of those accepted to medical school in Canada as of 2014. Depending on the medical school, schools in Canada admit those who speak English and French, and roughly 25% of all students accepted in Canada are native French speakers.

Foreign students are accepted into Canadian medical schools at low numbers, but many countries are represented. Commonly represented countries include Asia, Europe, Africa, the Caribbean, South America, Central America, Oceania, and North America. Statistically the greatest number of those accepted in 2014 came from China, India, Iran, and Germany. Attrition rates are very low Canada just as they are in the United States. Across Canada, less than 50 students on average withdrawal for any reason from all medical schools combined. Of these, approximately 60% are women. The average age for students graduating medical school in Canada is 26 years of age. The graduation age of those speaking French is 24 and the average age for those graduating who speak English is 26.

ASSOCIATION OF FACULTIES OF MEDICINE OF CANADA (AFMC)

The Association of Faculties of Medicine of Canada (AFMC) is the official organization representing all seventeen medical schools in Canada. The AFMC was formed in 1943 as the voice of academic medical education in Canada. Canada, through the AFMC, graduates over 2,800 physicians each year with over 12,000 active medical residents in training each year as well. AFMC provides guidance on undergraduate, graduate, and postgraduate education through several standing committees and resource groups. Issues such as student affairs, professionalism, global health, and diversity in medical school training are led by the AFMC. The AFMC states that medical schools have the obligation to "direct their education, research, and service activities towards addressing the priority health concerns of the community, region, and/or nation they have a mandate to serve." Multiple advocacy initiatives are championed to keep health and educational issues high on the agenda of the government.

Members of the AFMC serve, in part, along with representatives of the Canadian Medical Association (CMA) as members of the Committee on Accreditation of Canadian Medical Schools (CACMS). The CACMS accredits the medical education programs at all seventeen medical schools across Canada. Accreditation takes place with the Liaison Committee on Medical Education (LCME) in the United States. The AFMC participates in the accreditation of the Continuing Medical Educational programs as well. The AFMC also serves as the secretariat for the Canadian Conference on Medical Education and has done so since 2005. Using a process called the Interim Accreditation Review Process; the AFMC evaluates compliance with accreditation standards.

The AFMC utilizes two research and data divisions to aid in gathering and understanding postgraduate medical education in Canada. The Office of Research and Information Services (ORIS) and the Canadian Post-M.D. Education Registry (CAPER) maintain the largest collection of medical education data in Canada. Both of these divisions publish annual statistics which assist medical school students and applicants. Both organizations also support research initiatives across Canada.

AMERICAN MEDICAL RESIDENCY CERTIFICATION BOARD® (AMRCB®)

The AMRCB® provides certification for international medical students and graduates who desire a residency position in Canada and the United States. The AMRCB® also provides certification for Medical and Dental Schools located in the international community outside of Canada and the United States. The AMRCB® is not directly related to the accreditation process of medical schools in Canada. In conjunction with ECFMG® certification, both certifications recognize the qualitative and quantitative aspects of each student.

MEDICAL SCHOOL ACCREDITATION

The Committee on Accreditation of Canadian Medical Schools (CACMS) works in conjunction with the Liaison Committee on Medical Education (LCME) in the United States to ensure that each medical school located in Canada meets and maintains a quality medical education. Formal accreditation is required for medical schools to operate in Canada. Each medical school undergoes an on-site evaluation which covers multiple areas by a team of surveyors.

CACMS was formed in 1979 with the Canadian Medical Association and the Association of Canadian Medical Colleges (ACME). Canadian participation with the LCME was active prior to CACMS being formed. Canada and the United States have enjoyed a long standing cooperation in the area of medical education. Only Canadian schools accredited by CACMS are listed in the WHO/IMED world directory of medical schools.

CACMS describes the accreditation standards in the following categories:

1. Mission, Planning, Organization, and Integrity
2. Leadership and Administration
3. Academic and Learning Environments
4. Faculty Preparation, Productivity, Participation, and Policies
5. Educational Resources and Infrastructure
6. Competencies, Curricular Objectives, and Curricular Design
7. Curricular Content
8. Curricular Management, Evaluation, and Enhancement
9. Teaching, Supervision, Assessment, and Student and Patient Safety
10. Medical Student Selection, Assignment, and Progress
11. Medical Student Academic Support, Career Advising, and Educational Records
12. Medical Student Health Services, Personal Counseling, and Financial Aid Services

CHOOSING A MEDICAL CAREER

Once a student has decided that they may want to go to medical school, a large amount of work is needed to understand the application and interview process, the educational experience, and what is necessary in securing a medical residency in order to become a fully licensed physician. Many factors come into play to help shape the desire to pursue a career in medicine. Medicine can be a fulfilling and exciting career and also allows for financial stability. In addition, many different specialties and career paths exist in medicine to include clinical care, management, research, and teaching. According to the AAMC, approximately 60% of medical students plan to practice clinically, 10% desire teaching and research, and the remaining 30% are either undecided or have alternative plans.

Table 1.1: Decision on Pursuing a Career in Medicine

Time	Percent
Before High School	20%
During High School or Before College	29%
During the First Two Years of College	24%
During the Junior Year of College	11%
During the Senior Year of College	4%
After Completion of a Baccalaureate Degree	10%
After Completion of an Advanced Degree	2%

Source: AAMC's 2010 Matriculating Student Questionnaire (MSQ)

The specialties chosen by medical school graduates are diverse as well. Careers are available to those who like to problem solve, work with their hands, work primarily with their intellect, and varying combinations of these skills. Some students are attracted to primary or general care, while some are attracted to specific surgical specialties. Specialty choices can be impacted as well by the desire to live in a rural or city environment. For example, a student desiring to become a radiation oncologist and who desires to live in a rural environment, would have a mismatch that would not allow both to be realistic options. While the supply and demand of specific specialties may vary, in general, a projected shortage of nearly 100,000 physicians overall is expected in the U.S. and Canada by 2020.

Table 1.2: Specialty Consideration of Matriculating Medical Students

Specialty Consideration	Percentage
Internal Medicine	17.7
Pediatrics	13.7
Orthopedic Surgery	8.7
Emergency Medicine	8.5
Family Practice	7.9
OB/GYN	4.9
Neurology	4.4
Radiology	3.3
Dermatology	3.0
Anesthesiology	3.0
Ophthalmology	2.5

Source: AAMC's 2010 Matriculating Student Questionnaire (MSQ)

CHAPTER 2
MEDICAL SCHOOL ADMISSIONS REQUIREMENTS

Medical schools in Canada provide instruction over either three or four years. Although most students who are accepted into medical schools have already completed an undergraduate degree, the medical education in Canada is considered to be an undergraduate degree. Medical schools award either a Doctor of Medicine (MD) or a MDCM degree. The MDCM degree is Latin for *Medicinae Doctor et Chirurgiae Magister* which means "doctor of medicine and master of surgery."

Most students that enter medical school have completed a baccalaureate degree prior to beginning their medical studies. Although any field of study may be considered and accepted, the majority of students have completed a degree in the biological sciences. Most medical schools require the completion of a baccalaureate degree although not all do. Medical schools in Quebec allow students to begin medical studies after a two year Collège d'enseignement général et professionnel (CEGEP) diploma. Schools in Western Canada may accept students with only two years of college study, and schools in Ontario may accept students who have completed only three years of prior study.

Specific information on each school is listed individually, but on average, less than 10% of those applying to the positions in Canada each year are accepted. Tuition costs are less than $13,000 CAD on average for medical schools located outside of Quebec. In Quebec, average tuition is less than $3,000 CAD each year.

Specific medical schools will have individual requirements and individual expectations of students who are selected, but many generalities of accepted students remain constant. Undergraduate coursework, overall Grade Point Average (GPA) and individual science Grade Point Averages, MCAT® scores, and a quality personal statement are required in order to be considered for an interview. However, not every school in Canada requires the MCAT® for consideration. Primarily the schools that provide instruction in French do not require the MCAT® as there is currently no French equivalent to the MCAT®. Many schools have overall cut-off scores and segment cut-off scores on the MCAT® which must be met in order for consideration. A higher score on undergraduate grades and on the MCAT® will only help an applicant's chance of acceptance.

Admissions requirements for medical schools in Canada and the United States are generally the same. Each individual medical school may have specific courses or subtle variations in prerequisite coursework, thus applicants should specifically review requirements at each individual institution that they are considering applying to. Many handbooks are available allowing for reference for specific universities. Specific information for each Canadian medical school is listed with the individual school entry in the second half of this publication. General admission requirements should be understood by applicants as they prepare for a career in medicine. Admission criteria for medical schools in Canada and the United States are much stricter and detailed in comparison with many international medical schools.

GENERAL MEDICAL ADMISSIONS REQUIRMENTS

- Citizenship or permanent residency status
- Residence in a specific province or state (may allow preference in selection)
- A minimum of 90 credit hours of prerequisite coursework or a 4-year undergraduate degree from an accredited university or college
- Criminal records check
- Application fee
- Minimum Grade Point Average (GPA) of 3.0 or higher. In general, very high GPA's in the range of 3.75 or higher are required. Individual science GPA's may be required as well and are generally expected to be greater than 3.5.
- Medical College Admissions Test (MCAT®) scores. Scores are generally expected to be 8-10 in each individual section. MCAT® scores should have been achieved within the last three to five years.
- Prerequisite coursework to include the following:
  o English or French (dependent on language of instruction of the medical school) – two academic courses (6 semester hours)
  o General Biology – two academic courses with laboratories (6 semester hours)
  o General Physics – two academic courses with laboratories (6 semester hours)
  o General Chemistry – one academic year with laboratories (9 semester credits)
  o Organic Chemistry – one academic year with laboratories (9 semester credits)
  o Biochemistry – one or two academic courses with laboratories

Table: 2.1: Prerequisite Coursework Required by Two or More Canadian Medical Schools

Prerequisite Course Requirement	Number of Schools
Organic Chemistry	8
Inorganic Chemistry	7
Biology	7
Biochemistry	6
Physics	6
College English	4
College Mathematics	3
Humanities	3
Calculus	2
Social Sciences	2

Source: Medical School Admission Requirements (MSAR®), 2012-2013. AAMC

Table 2.2: Canadian Medical Schools that Require the MCAT®

MCAT® Required	MCAT® Not Required
University of Alberta Faculty of Medicine and Dentistry	University of Sherbrook Faculty of Medicine
University of British Columbia Faculty of Medicine	University de Montreal Faculty of Medicine
University of Calgary Faculty of Medicine	Laval University Faculty of Medicine
Dalhousie University Faculty of Medicine	Northern Ontario School of Medicine
University of Manitoba Faculty of Medicine	University of Ottawa Faculty of Medicine
McMaster University, Michael G. DeGroote School of Medicine	McGill University Faculty of Medicine**
Memorial University of Newfoundland Faculty of Medicine	
Queens University Faculty of Health Sciences	** The MCAT® is required for out-of-province and international applicants whose undergraduate training was completed outside of Canada
University of Saskatchewan College of Medicine	
University of Toronto Faculty of Medicine	
Western University, Schulich School of Medicine and Dentistry	

In addition, medical school applicants are expected to have solid letters of reference written by professors and/or physicians who know the applicant and who have had direct experience with the applicant. Students are expected to have valid, valuable, and verifiable extra-curricular activities and volunteer experiences. Personal essays are required and attention to detail is expected as is impeccable grammar. Applicants should describe their background and be able to coherently explain why they desire to pursue a career in medicine. In general, students are expected to have maintained a full-time academic schedule during their undergraduate career although individual circumstances are considered for those applicants who have undergone a part-time academic schedule.

In general, it is recommended that applicants apply to more than one medical school. An applicant's chance of selection will increase when several schools are applied to, and students who apply to only one school have the lowest statistical chances of acceptance. Applicants may have an advantage at specific institutions as well based on citizenship and geographic location of residence. Applicants should meet all prerequisites prior to applying and must ensure that internal deadlines are followed at each school.

Table 2.3: Methods of Preparing for Medical School Applications

Method	Percentage
Working or Volunteering in the Health Field	92.8%
MCAT® Preparation Course	65.3%
Laboratory Research	57.8%
Summer Enrichment Program	12.4%
Post-Baccalaureate Program to Complete Prerequisite Requirements	8.4%
Post-Baccalaureate Programs to Strengthen Academic Skills	5.9%

Source: AAMC's 2010 Matriculating Student Questionnaire (MSQ)

MEDICAL SCHOOL CURRICULUM

Individual medical schools have individual variations in curriculum, but overall, the majority of what is taught to medical students across Canada is the same. Even in the schools whose curriculum runs over three years instead of four, the curriculum is basically the same as four year schools. Three-year schools generally provide instruction uninterrupted over the summer. The first two years (or half) of the medical curriculum provides instruction on the basic sciences. The basic sciences include anatomy, biology, epidemiology, ethics, genetics, microbiology, pharmacology, and physiology. Some schools provide instruction in traditional lecture format while others base their educational program on organ systems. Many programs integrate problem-based learning as well into the curriculum. Laboratory work, simulated patient experiences, and introductory clinical experiences are used at all location during the basic science education.

The last two years (or second half) of medical school involves clinical rotations called clerkships. Clerkships provide the clinical training required to become a skilled and knowledgeable physician. Clerkships are supervised by physician instructors and resident physicians. Clerkship rotations include required rotations which are generally Internal Medicine, Family Medicine, Obstetrics and Gynecology, Pediatrics, Psychiatry. and Surgery. Emergency medicine is required by many schools as well. Elective rotations are required in the last year of study which can be in any interest of the student, although specific guidelines and direction are often required. Elective and required rotations allow a student to not only become knowledgeable in the various areas of medicine, but allow students to explore which area of medicine may be of interest to them. Some programs exist as well that allow students to obtain a dual degree such as a MBA or Ph.D.

Students in Canada take the Medical Council of Canada Qualifying Examination (MCCQE) during their final year of medical school. The MCCQE is administered by the Medical Council of Canada. This test is a multiple-choice, part short-answer computer examination. Students take Part II of the MCCQE which is an objective structured clinical examination after one year of residency training. Students are not eligible for licensing in Canada until they have completed both parts of the MCCQE (or the Certification Examination in Family Medicine). Students must pass board examination in their specialties in order to practice independently and do so generally in their last years of residency training. Depending on specialty, this is either conducted by the Royal College of Physicians and Surgeons of Canada (RCPSC) or the College of Family Physicians of Canada (CFPC). More information on licensure requirements is found in chapter seven.

FOREIGN APPLICANTS

For applicants to Canadian medical schools who are not Canadian citizens, specific understanding of the requirements of each school must be researched. Not all medical schools in Canada accept applications from foreign students. Some Canadian medical schools, however, have contracts with foreign institutions or governments to accept applications for positions. Canadian medical schools who participate in this may receive full compensation for those student positions. Often, these foreign students study in Canada during medical school and then return to their home country immediately thereafter for postgraduate training. Foreign students who train in Canada must obtain all required students authorizations and a student visa to enter Canada for the purpose of medical school study. Foreign students in Canada also pay a considerably higher rate for the education each year than their Canadian counterparts.

NON-TRADITIONAL APPLICANTS

Non-traditional applicants to medical schools are generally considered to be applicants who are older than 25, and/or those who have had prior careers or completed the educational process in a different educational discipline. While 50% of applicants aged 21-23 are accepted into medical school, only 25% of those ages 25-37 are accepted. Age is not, in general, a discriminating factor, and can, in fact, be a positive factor for some applicants. Overall, however, non-traditional applicants must be able to demonstrate solid academic success and have a high GPA and high MCAT® scores. It is important for applicants to demonstrate success in recent coursework, and not just in coursework taken many years back during their original course of study.

Non-traditional applicants must meet the same prerequisite qualifications as traditional applicants. It is understood, though, that the educational process will likely involve night-classes, community college courses, and part-time college enrollment as non-traditional applicants are often balancing a career and many times a family. Some prerequisite coursework may have been completed in a post-baccalaureate program as well. This is acceptable, although post-baccalaureate programs are not generally accredited but do offer the necessary prerequisite coursework. Some post-baccalaureate programs apply the coursework taken towards a Master's degree program. Some post-baccalaureate programs have a "feeder" relationship with a medical school that allows students to gain entry directly into medical school if a certain GPA is maintained during the coursework. Even though this relationship may be in place, the interview process is still required for all applicants.

REPEAT APPLICATIONS

For any student who is reapplying after not gaining acceptance during a prior year, they must work to understand what variables were involved that resulted in them not gaining acceptance. Objective data and feedback is the most useful tool. It is very likely that the numbers of qualified applicants simply overwhelmed the available spots as happens each year. It is equally as possible, though, that specific academic, professional, or personal qualities may have played a part in the applicant not being accepted. Repeat applicants by students are often successful in subsequent years.

Chapter 3
The Application Process

The application process to medical school can be complicated, and unlike in the United States, the application process to Canadian medical schools varies by school and province. Many factors are important in the application selection process. Many schools rely heavily on the interview for selections, but it is the academic details in the application that enable students to be selected for the interview. The "average matched medical school applicant" has the following academic criteria: Overall GPA of 3.8, Science GPA of 3.31, a Non-Science GPA of 3.75, and an average MCAT® score of 31.2. Average MCAT® sub-scores of accepted applicants are a Verbal Reasoning score of 9.8, a Physical Science score of 10.5, a Biological Science score of 10.9, and a Q on the writing sample when applicable.

The personal qualities of the individual applicants are extremely important as well in the selection process, but an applicant is not able to demonstrate these in an interview if the academic history is not competitive enough to illicit an actual interview. Other student experiences such as research, prior leadership, volunteer activities, letters of recommendation, and extracurricular activities are important as well. Applicants should remember that despite the high overall qualifications of selected applicants that these are average scores, and many students are selected each year for medical school with academic records well below the actual average.

Canadian medical schools select applicants nearly entirely based on Canadian citizenship or residency and province of residency; landed immigrant status; or those with an active Canadian visa. Several schools do allow for a small number of other applicants to apply from the United States and the international community. In addition, special consideration is given to aboriginal Canadians and applicants who are in the Canadian armed forces at many institutions. Application deadlines will vary by medical school.

Letters of recommendations will be required. Students are most often required to have two to five letters of recommendations forwarded to the individual schools. Several schools request a specific number of recommendations only, and a student should send only the number requested. Of the letters of recommendation, letters are often required from science faculty, advisors, and pre-medical committees if the student's school has one of these.

Do not assume that all material and items sent to the schools have been received. A student should, using care not to be overbearing, call and check that items have arrived at the schools and that their file is complete and the application is being processed. Countless students have been disqualified from applying after the application deadline has passed simply because a transcript or letter of recommendation was never sent, lost in the mail, or misplaced by the school. Once the application is complete, each school will individually contact the students that they are interested in to schedule an interview.

Older, non-traditional students are often apprehensive about applying to medical school. This concern is unfounded, as non-traditional students are found in large numbers throughout the Canadian system. Canadian medical schools often seek students who are mature and who have had many life experiences. The skills that non-traditional students bring to medical school are often appreciated and valued by the medical schools.

MCAT®

The Medical College Admissions Test (MCAT®) is arguably the most difficult standardized test that any student will attempt in any discipline. The MCAT® has been offered for over 80 years and is now offered over 30 times each year at multiple locations in the U.S, Canada, and internationally, where it had previously been offered only twice a year. This author strongly recommends that applicants take the MCAT® in the spring of their junior year so that if they are dissatisfied with their test scores, they can retake it again later in the year. An applicant's knowledge of the sciences in general biology, general inorganic chemistry, organic chemistry, and general physics is tested. The overall content is tested with multiple-choice questions and is divided over three scored, and one un-scored section. Overall reading comprehension and quantitative reasoning are also assessed. A student's writing abilities are still currently tested, although this is currently being revised and will no longer be included in the near future.

Except for rare exceptions, the MCAT® is required by all medical schools in Canada and the U.S. and is used and/or required by many international medical schools. The MCAT® is often used by other graduate and health professional programs as well and is currently taken by over 85,000 students each year. Successful completion of the MCAT® is currently identified as a key to future success in medicine. The overarching goal is to assess a student's problem solving and critical thinking skills.

The MCAT® is currently undergoing major revisions currently in 2015. The MCAT® is standardized and is offered in a multiple-choice format so that all students can be evaluated using the same criteria. The Association of American Medical Colleges (AAMC) contracts with physicians, undergraduate university faculty, medical school faculty, and other experts to develop the test each year. The MCAT® underwent changes in 1991 so that the MCAT® of today is significantly different and includes more passages concerning the humanities and the social sciences than were previously available.

During each testing session, multiple versions of the MCAT® are given. Many of the passages students will receive will be the same, but several will be completely different. Although there will be content differences from test to test, the principles being tested are the same. No notes, calculators, or outside sources are permitted to be used during the testing. Total time to take the test, including breaks, is just over five hours.

The MCAT® currently consists of four sections, which are the Physical Sciences, Biological Sciences, Verbal Reasoning, and either the current Writing Sample or the new Trial Section depending on when the test is taken. All students who are preparing to apply to a health professions school are eligible to take the MCAT® which includes: Allopathic, Podiatric, Osteopathic, and Veterinary medicine. Students will be asked to accept a statement that verifies they are taking the exam only for the purpose of applying to a health professions school. Students who are currently enrolled in a medical school or those not planning on applying to a health professions school will require special permission to take the test. The requirements to be eligible to take the test are the same for U.S., Canadian, and international medical students.

Prospective MCAT® applicants will be required to have an ID, user name, and password in order to register for the examination. The current cost of the examination is dependent upon when a student registers and if they are eligible for fee assistance. Fee assistance is designed for applicants who would not be able to take the examination or apply to medical school without this assistance. Those eligible for fee assistance also get a free copy of the Official Guide to the MCAT® Exam, and access to The Official MCAT® Self-Assessment Package.

For those applying without fee assistance greater than one month before the exam, the cost is $330 CAD with a $78 CAD fee to reschedule. For students applying two to three weeks prior the exam without fee assistance, the cost is $330 CAD and a $150 CAD fee to reschedule. Applicants who apply one to two weeks prior to the exam without fee assistance are charged $391 CAD and are not eligible to reschedule at a lower fee. For those who are eligible for fee assistance and apply greater than one month before the exam, the cost is $120 CAD with a $30 CAD fee to reschedule. For students applying two to three weeks prior the exam with fee assistance, the cost is $120 CAD and a $54 CAD fee to reschedule. Applicants who apply one to two weeks prior to the exam with fee assistance are charged $180 CAD and are not eligible to reschedule at a lower fee.

The exam will be given in order starting with the Physical Sciences, followed by Verbal Reasoning, Biological Sciences, and finally the current writing sample or the new Trial Section. The grading design is being changed to reflect a range of 1 to 15 for each section which will then be converted overall to a score ranging from 1 to 15 as well. The lowest score is reflected with a one and the highest score is a fifteen.

The Physical Sciences section is constructed so that information learned in the first year courses of general physics and general inorganic chemistry is tested. The physics tested is not calculus based. This section of the MCAT® is given in 70 minutes, consists of 52 questions, and covers passage-based questions and non-passage-based questions. The scientific information is presented in passages, charts, graphs, and tables. Scientific problem solving is emphasized as is the interpretation of data. The questions given are generally 50% physics related and 50% chemistry related, but this can vary with each individual test and over individual years. Some MCAT® scores have been distributed by as much as 70/30 on these topics.

The Verbal Reasoning section is constructed so that the critical thinking, comprehension, and reasoning abilities of the applicant are tested. This section of the MCAT® is given over 60 minutes and consists of 40 questions. All of the questions in this section are passage-based. The passages can contain information about virtually any subject matter to include the social sciences and the humanities as well as the physical sciences. Knowledge of specific subjects is not a prerequisite because all of the answers can be found in, or gleaned from, the passages.

The Biological Sciences section is presented in much the same manner as the Physical Sciences. This section of the test is constructed so that information learned in the first year courses of general biology and organic chemistry is tested. This section is also given over a 70 minute period, consists of 52 questions, and covers passage-based and non-passage-based questions. This information is presented with passages, charts, graphs, and tables. The subject matter tested is usually distributed 50/50 on biology and organic chemistry questions, but this is also variable.

The Trial Section is currently an un-scored section and will consist of 32 questions and will be given over 45 minutes. This section is voluntary and those who choose to take it currently will receive compensation. It is the last section tested during the exam. The Trial Section will consist of questions in biochemistry, biology, chemistry, and physics; or in biology, psychology, and sociology. Questions in the Trial Section are generated based on responses given earlier in the exam.

The Writing Sample section will no longer be included as part of the MCAT® in 2015. In place of the Writing Sample, the current voluntary un-scored Trial Section is being used which initially began in 2013. The Writing Sample was constructed so that the students would complete two separate handwritten essays. Both essays had to be completed within 60 minutes, with each essay being completed individually within 30 minutes. This process was designed so that students could display their proficiency in writing and in their analytical skills. The essay topics did not require any prerequisite knowledge of subject matter and related to virtually any subject. Subjects that were sensitive, emotional, or offensive were not included in the essay topics.

Students will have the option on test day to release their scores to specific schools or to have their scores voided. The scores for the Biological, Physical, and Verbal sections are given on a range of 1 to 15. The scores of all students who take the MCAT® are processed. The scores are distributed basically along a parabolic curve so that only a few of the students who score poorly will receive 1's, and only a few of those who have perfect scores will receive 15's. The Writing Sample was scored on a range from "J" through "T". Each individual essay was graded on a range from 1-6 with a maximum of 12 total points available. A "J" resulted from receiving 1 point, a "K" from receiving 2 points, and so on. The highest score, a "T", was achieved by receiving 11 or 12 points. Students are able to retake the exam if they are not satisfied with the scores that they achieve, and many students choose to take a preparatory course in order to adequately prepare for the test.

Students often wonder what MCAT® scores are needed to gain acceptance into medical school. This is often difficult to determine as admissions criteria vary from year to year and for each individual medical school. The MCAT® scores are only a part of the total application, but they are most often a large part. Admissions committees will use these scores to determine which applicants will succeed in not only their university's curriculum, but prospectively on the USMLE® licensing exams as well. Each school will have their own methodology of evaluating MCAT® scores. Some schools will consider the highest set of scores, some will use the highest score in each testing area, some will average all the scores, and some will weigh all scores equally. The MCAT® is just one part of the overall application one uses to apply to medical school. Other factors include the overall and science grade point averages (GPA's); letters of recommendation; the medical school interview; the difficulty and breadth of the undergraduate education; extracurricular activities; overall attitude and diversity; personal statements; and work, research, and volunteer related medical activities. Scores on the Verbal and the Science sections will usually need to be in the range of 7-10 to gain acceptance. Writing Sample scores usually need to be in the range of an "O" to gain acceptance. This is not, however, always the case. Students with overall scores in the low 20's and with writing scores of "L's" and "M's" are accepted every year. Many schools have MCAT® cutoff scores that a student must meet in order to apply. Cutoff scores are usually in the mid-20's and writing cutoff scores are often set at an "M" or an "O".

The bottom line is that although a low MCAT® score will not prevent a solid applicant from gaining acceptance into medical school, a very high MCAT® score can nearly cement a place for the well-rounded student. It is of paramount importance for prospective applicants to study for and to take the MCAT® very seriously. Higher scores can result in higher degrees of success.

Table 3.1: Matriculating Student Preparation to Retake the MCAT®

Method of Preparation	Percentage
Change in Study Habits	39.1%
Online MCAT Practice Examinations	25.3%
MCAT Preparation Course	12.6%
Completing Additional Coursework	7.4%
Private Tutoring	1.9%
Seeking Advice from Mentor/Advisor	1.1%

Source: AAMC's 2010 Matriculating Student Questionnaire (MSQ)

PERSONAL STATEMENT

The personal statement that is presented on the application is very important. This statement is the opportunity for the prospective student to state their reasons for seeking a degree in medicine, as well as any other reasons that the student may feel are important to include. This will be the primary opportunity for medical schools to evaluate the applicant's writing proficiency, intelligence, motivation, thoroughness, and overall reasons for pursuing medicine. Students should take their time creating this statement and spend as much time on this as on any other part of the application process. The personal statement should be read, proofread, perfected, and reread. The statement should be read by as many persons as possible such as family members, friends, professors, and college staff if possible. Any grammatical mistakes or miswording will reflect extremely poorly on the applicant. Medical schools in Canada are not looking for students who are sloppy, careless, or do not take the proper time to effectively complete a written document.

The personal statement should reflect the reasons the student is pursuing medicine. Countless students have produced eloquent displays of grammatical perfection that stated nothing about why they wanted to become a physician. Canadian medical schools want to know why you want to be a physician; do not leave this out. Students often choose to tell a story, use quotations, and to weave intricate personal descriptions into their personal statements. This is fine. A poignant description of a personal tragedy, the death of a loved one, or the humanistic issues witnessed during volunteer or work experiences may give the applicant depth. Uniqueness and interesting statements will also catch the attention of the admissions board and may weigh in the student's favor. The student should be sure that the statement is cohesive, complete, and clearly describes the applicant. The difference in the personal statements of accepted medical students is extensive, but the common thread throughout is clarity and well-crafted writing.

Personal statements generally follow three themes. The first is the "Life History" approach. The focuses on significant life events that have shaped the applicants and helped them to form the desire to become a physician should be included. What is difficult about this approach is maintaining a clear timeline and cohesive story throughout. The second approach is "Telling a Story." This approach builds the personal statement on a particular, often life-changing or life-affirming event. This style of essay is often one of the most effective ones and is more easily remembered than other models. A story is easier for the Admissions Committee members to read and defines reasonably easily who the applicant is. The final approach that is often used is the "History in School" approach. This focuses on the educational journey of the applicant and can work well for those with high academic qualifications as this can highlight aspects that separate the applicant from other applicants. This approach also allows students to demonstrate their strengths with specific examples. The key for success in this approach is to connect the academic successes with one's overall goals

APPLICANT CLASSIFICATION

Applicants to Canadian medical schools will be classified as applicants from the North American system of education, the British system of education, or from all other systems of education. This classification will determine what specific requirements must be met in order to qualify for admission. Applicants from the North American system of education are considered applicants from the United States and Canada. Applicants from the British system of education must possess a strong science background. All other applicants will include those from any country other than the United States, Canada, and Great Britain. Applicants from countries with similar educational standards as are present in Canada, and those from countries with variations from these Canadian standards, will be evaluated individually by the Admissions Committees of each school. Each applicant should meet the educational requirements for admission to medical school in their home country.

Any applicant whose native language is not English will usually be required to take and pass the Test of English as a Foreign Language (TOEFL®) or the International English Language Testing System (IELTS™) for schools that provide instruction in English. Acceptable pass ranges may vary by institution, but in general, acceptable minimum scores on the TOEFL® are 600 (paper-based), 250 (computer-based), or 100 (internet-based). For the IELTS™ the general minimum passing score is 7.0 overall. Canadian medical schools that provide instruction in French will require fluency in French in order for an applicant to be considered for admission.

APPLICATION SERVICES

AMERICAN MEDICAL COLLEGES APPLICATION SERVICE (AMCAS®)

The American Medical Colleges Application Service (AMCAS®) is a centralized medical school application processing service that is operated by the Association of Medical Colleges. Nearly all medical schools in the United States (expect for those located in Texas) and Puerto Rico use this service. At this time, no medical schools in Canada are utilizing the AMCAS® service. Some medical schools use the AMCAS® as the only required application, while others use it as the initial application and subsequently require a secondary application. AMCAS® is only available for pre-medical students applying to the first year entering class at participating medical schools. Any student interested in Advanced Standing or transferring into a medical school from another medical school must contact the individual schools for process information. The AMCAS® process is not involved in the selection process and does not offer advice on applying to medical schools. The application fee as of 2016 is $192 CAD for the first medical school applied to and $44 CAD for each subsequent medical school.

AMCAS® allows students to send in reference letters and other application materials such as undergraduate and AMRCB® educational transcripts which are subsequently sent in a complete application to each medical school applied to. The AMCAS® website also provides additional information on issues such as opportunities for fellowships, transitioning to the work force, debt management, and other information. United States osteopathic medical schools have a similar application system called the American Association of Colleges of Osteopathic Medicine Application Service (AACOMAS).

The AMCAS® application is submitted online. Application deadlines are absolute including application for early decision. Once all information has been received, AMCAS® processes the application and assigns a verified AMCAS® GPA. GPA's are calculated for Biology, Chemistry, Physics, and Mathematics (BCPM GPA); and for All Other classes (AO GPA). The entire process of verification takes up to six weeks. The peak time for applications is June through September each year. Applications received during this time period can take longer to process. All applications are required to include the following: all academic transcripts and descriptions of all work and extracurricular activities; letters of recommendation; legal history; a personal statement; and MCAT® and/or other scores such as GMAT/LSAT/GRE scores. The reason most applications are delayed is that students have not submitted each and every transcript from every school that they have attended, regardless if they received academic credit or not. Once completed, the AMCAS® application will be sent to all medical schools that were designated by the candidate.

ONTARIO MEDICAL SCHOOL APPLICATION SERVICE (OMSAS)

All six schools located in Ontario utilize the Ontario Medical School Application Service (OMSAS). OMSAS is a centralized application service that serves McMaster University, Northern Ontario School of Medicine, Queen's University, University of Toronto, University of Ottawa, and Western University. OMSAS allows applicants to submit only one application and set of application materials which can be delivered to any number of the schools located in Ontario. This application is independently assessed by each institution and OMSAS has no bearing on acceptance and does not operate like a matching service where numbers of interviews are controlled through the system.

The OMSAS application opens up in mid-July. The application process and admission requirements for each school of medicine located in Ontario are found on this site. The OMSAS application fee is $210 CAD and each school has a supplementary application fee as well for each school applied to with a cost ranging from $75-115 CAD.

Students must register for an account beginning in mid-September each year with October 1st being the deadline to have created the account for that application year. Payments for the applications must be made generally within two days after the deadline. Payments are accepted by online banking and Western Union Banking Solutions. International payments are accepted by bank-to-bank transfers only. For medical schools that require the MCAT®, scores must have been submitted by November 1st of the application year. Offers for admission start in May of the following year. Final student transcripts must be received by the end of June.

Table 3.2: Individual University Application Fees in addition to OMSAS Fees

Medical School	Application Fee*
McMaster University	$115
Northern Ontario School of Medicine	$85
Queen's University	$100
University of Toronto	$110
University of Ottawa	$75
Western University	$100

Source: Admission Requirements of Canadian Faculties of Medicine

*All funds in Canadian Funds

OMSAS Contact Information:

Ontario Universities Application Centre

170 Research Lane

Guelph ON N1G 5E2

Tel: 519-823-1940

Fax: 519-823-5232

E-Mail: omsas@ouac.on.ca

Website: www.ouac.on.ca/omsas

SECONDARY APPLICATIONS

Several medical schools require a secondary application after the primary application has been reviewed. Some Canadian institutions send out secondary applications to all students who have applied, while others only send secondary applicants to students who are deemed as competitive. Often secondary applications are sent out for applicants who have MCAT® scores and grade point averages above a specific cutoff number. Cutoff numbers can vary each year, however, dependent upon the overall scores from the applicant pool for that specific year. Secondary applications usually are associated with another fee ranging from $50-150 CAD.

The content of secondary applications varies, but many ask specific questions that illicit short essay response. The response to these questions must be well thought out, professionally crafted, and proofread for any errors. Examples of questions that may be asked include

- Why do you want to practice medicine?

- What medical specialty are you interested in?

- Where do you see yourself in 5, 10, or 15 years?

- Give us examples of your leadership experience?

- What is your greatest success? What is your most significant failure?

- Who is your favorite historical person?

Chapter 4

The Interview

The interview process can be a major hurdle to overcome and will be the primary opportunity for individual students to demonstrate their value. Interviews with Canadian medical schools are conducted nearly exclusively in person, and regional interviews can occur in some cases. Although one interview is generally all that is required for most applicants, it may be necessary to have an additional interview in some cases. The policies and procedures for the interview process are usually provided for the applicants upon receipt of the initial application. The school's admission office can provide clarification of procedures if necessary.

Keep in mind that once the school grants an interview, that they have already made the decision that the applicant has the overall qualities that the school is looking for. The interview is often used to weed out unstable and immature applicants as well as to select the most impressive candidates. The goal is to sell yourself; applicants should therefore be prepared to make a good sales pitch. Medical schools in Canada understand that they are often competing for applicants with other Canadian and United States medical schools. Most interviews will be reasonably relaxed and interviewers generally do not have the goal of pinning applicants down. Any direct contact with a prospective school should be conducted in professional attire. Do not make the mistake of ever under-dressing.

An applicant should expect to be asked questions concerning their reasons for pursuing medicine and their personal and academic histories. The interview is also an opportunity to ask questions of the school which may be very important in choosing which school to attend. Be prepared to ask questions as this can show motivation and preparation, both of which are desirable qualities.

Applicants should be familiar with, and observe all, application procedures of the school and submit all necessary documents in a timely manner. The medical schools should be kept informed of any change of address or telephone number. Applicants should promptly respond to invitations for an interview and promptly notify the school immediately if the interview needs to be cancelled or rescheduled.

BEFORE THE INTERVIEW

Be Prepared - Do not go into the interview without having practiced. Mock interviews and well thought out answers will be extremely beneficial. Also, students should be up-to-date on current events as these questions are fair game. Newspapers and magazines will help applicants to prepare for these questions. It is particularly helpful to have researched information on the specific medical school, country, and region where the medical school is located.

Dress Professionally - The first impression that will be made will be the student's physical appearance. Men should dress in a dark suit with a tasteful tie and shined shoes. Suits should be black, blue, or gray and ties should not have any loud designs or colors. Women should wear dress coordinates or a suit, although a suit may not always be appropriate for all schools. Shoes should not have heels that are too high and make-up and jewelry should be tasteful. All students should have a leather binder with them for the information that they will receive.

Arrive Early - The absolute worst thing that a prospective student can do is to arrive late for an interview. All students should have several copies of their application and personal statement with them to hand out if requested and have reviewed these prior to arrival. Be familiar with the school catalog and with any programs of which the school is particularly proud. From the moment the student sets foot into the city they are interviewing in, they must treat everyone with the utmost respect. This applies particularly to the administrative staff and students of the school, because one never knows who the person they cut-off in the parking lot or were rude to at a restaurant may be. This may be one of the interviewers. One must also treat all support staff with respect, particularly the administrative and secretarial staff as they often will have direct input on prospective students, and are often vocal on the impressions they have of individual applicants.

DURING THE INTERVIEW

Be Self-Confident - Applicants should be self-confident but it no way pushy or overbearing. It is acceptable to be witty and charming, but not sarcastic. Often, the actual answer to a question is not nearly as important as the manner in which the question is handled. Poise and confidence will go a long way

Exhibit Control - Begin by acknowledging the interviewer by name, introduce yourself, and offer a handshake. Next, do not exhibit nervous movements. Fidgeting, talking too fast, shaking one's leg, or fondling a pen or brochure can be very irritating to the interviewer. Do not forget to maintain appropriate eye contact and to respond timely to comments or humor from the interviewer.

Answer Questions Intelligently - Think about what is going to be said before it is said. Stuttering or rambling while answering a question will cause the student to appear unintelligent. Do not answer questions with an attitude or like a know-it-all. Interviewers are not looking for students who know everything. If a student does not know an answer, they should say so. It will be much more beneficial to be honest than it will be to make something up and appear shallow and dishonest. If the interviewer wants to aggravate or antagonize the applicant, do not respond in the same manner. Stay calm and relaxed and understand that this is probably only a test to see how the applicant is going to react under stressful situations.

AFTER THE INTERVIEW

Remain Composed - After the interview, offer a handshake and say good-bye. Tell the interviewer that their time is appreciated. Be prepared to take a tour of the school and/or hospital. Composure during the tours and during lunch will be just as important as it is during the interview. The tour guides are usually medical school students and they may have input into the student's evaluation as well.

Send Thank-You Notes - Many students often skip this last step; do not be one of them. Sending thank-you notes gives the student one last chance to contact the school and to reiterate their interest and the desire to attend that school. Interviewers will appreciate this formality and it will help them to remember the student in a positive light. The best approach is to write the thank-you notes immediately after the interviews. Memories of the event, interactions, and specific content of individual discussions will fade over several hours to several days.

THE MULTIPLE MINI INTERVIEW (MMI)

The Multiple Mini Interview (MMI) is a series of short, structured interviews used to assess personal traits and qualities of applicants. Each mini interview provides an applicant with two minutes to read a question/scenario and to mentally prepare before entering the interview room. Upon entering, the applicant has eight minutes of dialogue with one or more interviewers/assessors. At the conclusion of the interview, the interviewer/assessor uses the next two-minute period to evaluate the applicant while the candidate moves to the next scenario. This pattern is repeated through a circuit of up to 10 stations taking up to 120 minutes (depending on the number of test stations). The MMI was derived from the well-known OSCE (Objective Structured Clinical Examination) used by most medical education programs to assess a student's application of clinical skills and knowledge (Eva *et al.* 2004a). The MMI differs from the OSCE in that the MMI is neither clinical nor objective.

The traditional interview has been replaced with the MMI for most Canadian medical schools for several reasons which include:

- The MMI allows multiple opportunities for insight into an applicant's abilities.

- The MMI dilutes the effect of examiner bias and chance.

- Applicants can feel confident they will be given a chance to recover from a bad experience at a station by moving to a new, independent reviewer.

- MMI stations can be structured so that all applicants respond to the same questions and interviewers receive background information directly.

- MMI stations can be designed with a great deal of flexibility to select students with the personal attributes desired.

- The MMI has been found to better predict pre-clerkship OSCE performance than assessment of non-academic traits by autobiographical submissions, a simulated tutorial, or the standard panel interview.

Personal attributes such as communication skills and maturity will be assessed at each individual MMI station. Station scenarios may be structured to specifically judge an applicant's ethical and critical decision-making abilities; commitment to help others; knowledge of the healthcare system; understanding of health determinants in a local or global context; desire to study medicine; or non-academic achievements. The MMI was developed initially at McMaster University in 2003 where it was initially used in parallel with the panel interview. McMaster Medical School has been using the MMI in selecting students since 2004 and has been used nearly universally in Canada since 2009. There appears to be a consensus building across the country that the MMI is the process of choice for assessing the non-cognitive abilities of medical school applicants.

PRACTICE MMI QUESTIONS

The following 10 descriptions of potential MMI stations are provided directly from materials generated from McMaster University.

Station 1: Placebo (Ethical Decision Making)^

Dr. Smith recommends homeopathic medicines to his patients. There is no scientific evidence or widely accepted theory to suggest that homeopathic medicines work, and Dr. Smith doesn't believe them to. He recommends homeopathic medicine to people with mild and non-specific symptoms such as fatigue, headaches and muscle aches, because he believes that it will do no harm, but will give them reassurance.

Consider the ethical problems that Dr. Smith's behavior might pose. Discuss these issues with the interviewer.

Station 2: Aspartame (Critical Thinking)^

A message that recently appeared on the Web warned readers of the dangers of aspartame (artificial sweetener – NutraSweet, Equal) as a cause of an epidemic of multiple sclerosis (a progressive chronic disease of the nervous system) and systemic lupus (a multisystem auto-immune disease). The biological explanation provided was that, at body temperature, aspartame releases wood alcohol (methanol), which turns into formic acid, which is in the same class of drugs as cyanide and arsenic. Formic acid, they argued, causes metabolic acidosis. Clinically, aspartame poisoning was argued to be a cause of joint pain, numbness, cramps, vertigo, headaches, depression, anxiety, slurred speech and blurred vision. The authors claimed that aspartame remains on the market because the food and drug industries have powerful lobbies in Congress. They quoted Dr. Russell Blaylock, who said, "The ingredients stimulate the neurons of the brain to death, causing brain damage of varying degrees."

Critique this message, in terms of the strength of the arguments presented and their logical consistency. Your critique might include an indication of the issues that you would like to delve into further before assessing the validity of these claims.

Station 3: Air Travel (Communication Skills)^

Your company needs both you and a co-worker (Sara, a colleague from another branch of the company) to attend a critical business meeting in New York. You have just arrived to drive Sara to the airport.

Sara is in the room.

Station 4: Deterrent Fees (Knowledge of the Health Care System)^

Recently, the Prime Minister of Canada raised the issue of deterrent fees (a small charge, say $10, which everyone who initiates a visit to a health professional would have to pay at the first contact) as a way to control health care costs. The assumption is that this will deter people from visiting their doctor for unnecessary reasons.

Consider the broad implications of this policy for health and health care costs. For example, do you think the approach will save health care costs? At what expense? Discuss this issue with the interviewer.

Station 5: Standard Interview 1^

Why do you want to be a physician? Discuss this question with the interviewer.

Station 6: Circumcision (Ethical Decision Making)^

The Canadian Pediatric Association has recommended that circumcisions "not be routinely performed". They base this recommendation on their determination that "the benefits have not been shown to clearly outweigh the risks and costs." Doctors have no obligation to refer for, or provide, a circumcision, but many do, even when they are clearly not medically necessary. Ontario Health Insurance Plan (OHIP) no longer pays for unnecessary circumcisions.

Consider the ethical problems that exist in this case. Discuss these issues with the interviewer.

Station 7: Class Size (Critical Thinking)^

Universities are commonly faced with the complicated task of balancing the educational needs of their students and the cost required to provide learning resources to a large number of individuals. As a result of this tension, there has been much debate regarding the optimal size of classes. One side argues that smaller classes provide a more educationally effective setting for students, while others argue that it makes no difference, so larger classes should be used to minimize the number of instructors required.

Discuss your opinion on this issue with the examiner.

Station 8: Parking Garage (Communication Skills)^

The parking garage at your place of work has assigned parking spots. On leaving your spot, you are observed by the garage attendant as you back into a neighboring car, a BMW, knocking out its left front headlight and denting the left front fender. The garage attendant gives you the name and office number of the owner of the neighboring car, telling you that he is calling ahead to the car owner Mike. The garage attendant tells you that Mike is expecting your visit.

Enter Mike's office.

Station 9: Preferential Admission (Knowledge of the Health Care System)^

Due to the shortage of physicians in rural communities such as those in Northern Ontario, it has been suggested that medical programs preferentially admit students who are willing to commit to a 2- or 3-year tenure in an under-serviced area upon graduation.

Consider the broad implications of this policy for health and health care costs. For example, do you think the approach will be effective? At what expense? Discuss this issue with the interviewer.

Station 10: Standard Interview 2^

What experiences have you had (and what insights have you gained from these experiences) that lead you to believe you would be a good physician?

Discuss this question with the interviewer.

^*The descriptions of the 10 stations above were provided directly from materials generated by McMaster University*

POSSIBLE INTERVIEW QUESTIONS

- How are you today? Did you have trouble locating us?
- Why do you want to be a doctor?
- Which fields of medicine are you interested in?
- What kind of experiences do you have in the medical field?
- Where do you plan to practice medicine?
- What are your goals in medicine?
- Where do you see yourself in 5, 10, or 15 years?
- Why did you apply to our school?
- The future outlook of medicine is concerning. Why would you want to enter this field?
- Would you go to our program if I gave you an acceptance letter right now?
- Why should we choose you over all of the other applicants?
- What will you bring to the class if you are accepted?
- What other programs have you applied to besides ours?
- Did anyone you know influence your career choice?
- Do you have family members who are physicians?
- Were you influenced by a relative to pursue a career in medicine?
- Why are your qualifications any better or different than the other applicants?
- Tell us your definition of a professional.
- If you were held up at gunpoint with a loved one, what would you do?
- What do you think of affirmative action?
- Give me an example of something you did that was wrong.
- Explain you research project.
- Would you get out of your car in a highway to help an accident victim?
- Why is your MCAT® much higher/lower than your GPA?
- If an AIDS patient were bleeding profusely from an injury, what would you do?
- What do you think is the most difficult issue facing the medical community?
- What do you think of herbal or alternative medicine?
- What are your thoughts on the Accountable Care Act in the United States?
- What would you do if a family member decided to solely depend on alternative medicine for their treatment?
- How will you handle being taught something that you already know?
- Can you handle somebody throwing up on you?
- What are your thoughts on Medicare reform?
- What is the greatest problem facing medicine today?
- Can you afford to attend medical school?
- How would you improve preventive healthcare settings?
- What is the most embarrassing moment of your life?
- How would you improve access to healthcare in your country?
- How much alcohol do you drink?
- Do you feel that the government should be involved with mandating insurance?
- How would you control the rising cost of healthcare?
- Do you think horizontally or vertically?
- What interests do you have outside of medicine?
- How would a friend describe you?
- What is Preventive Medicine?
- Do you plan to continue your hobbies as you go through medical school?
- If you had one day to do anything, what would you do?
- What row in a classroom do you normally sit in and why?

- What was the last book that you read and would you recommend it?
- What was the last movie that you saw?
- What did you do in your last job?
- Can you define what hope is?
- When you die, what do you want your tombstone to say?
- What is the most important impact of medicine on humanity?
- How do your hobbies relate to being a physician?
- Do you think grade point averages are a fair way to evaluate students?
- If physicians were paid the same as teachers, would you still want to be a physician?
- Which classes did you enjoy the most and why?
- How would your friends describe your personality?
- Do you have an autocratic personality?
- How is your relationship with your parents?
- What is your opinion on animal research?
- What is a physician's role in the politics of abortion?
- What are your strengths and weaknesses?
- What one thing would you change about yourself?
- Is there something about you that would make you difficult to get along with?
- What type of people do you get along with well?
- Describe the most exciting event of your life.
- What do you think will be the most difficult aspect of medical school?
- Why did you do so poorly in _____ (a particular class)?
- Does racism still exist?
- Do you think that your classes were enough to prepare you for our program?
- Imagine that you find a lamp that gives you three wishes. What would they be?
- You discover that one of your peers is abusing drugs. What would you do?
- Should people have the right to sell their own organs?
- What qualities would you look for in your doctor?
- What qualities would you look for in your patients?
- Are your afraid of death?
- How do you tell a child that you have to amputate his arm?
- One of your letters of recommendation describes you as ___. Do you agree with that description?
- What would you do if a nurse refuses to carry out your orders?
- If you could be any animal, what would you be and why?
- If you could be any car, what would you be and why?
- Do you believe in life after death?
- Who do you admire the most in your life?
- If you could choose one figure in history to have dinner with, who would it be?
- Have you always put forth your best effort in every situation?
- Tell me about something that you know a lot about?
- You have just diagnosed a man with a sexually transmitted disease that he did not get from his wife. He says that he is not going to tell her. What would you do?
- If you find that the professor with whom you have done research has changed some of the data before publication, what would you do?
- During your clinical rotations, you treated a wealthy patient. He has decided to give you $100,000. What would you do with the money?
- What would you do if you saw a fellow medical student cheating on an exam?
- What role has stress played in your life?
- What are your thoughts on abortion?
- Describe your best friend.

- What are your thoughts on Euthanasia?
- How do you feel about fetal tissue research?
- How would you tell a patient that they have cancer?
- What would you do if your supervising doctor was under the influence of alcohol?
- A young teenager who is pregnant comes to you to discuss her options but says she has not told her parents about her pregnancy. How would you handle this?
- Do you think doctors are getting paid too much or too little?
- Do you think that decreasing the salaries of physicians can solve rising healthcare cost issues?
- What do you think about socialized medicine?
- What do you think of the doctor shortage/oversupply in different areas?
- What would you do if a doctor told you to give a medicine that you knew would harm the patient??
- Why do you think the number of applicants has been growing every year despite the problems we face in medicine?
- What would you do if you do not get into medical school this year?

QUESTIONS TO ASK

- What is the MCCQE pass rate on part 1 and part 2 for your school?
- Does your school offer, or require a MCCQE review course?
- What are specific problems you have seen in your students?
- Is your school certified by the AMRCB®?
- With which hospitals does your school have an affiliation?
- Is French/English widely spoken by the staff and patients I will work with?
- How are students chosen for clinical rotations in certain locations?
- What percentages of your graduates obtain a residency in Canada?
- What services are available for students who are struggling academically?
- What services are available for students struggling socially?
- What services are available for students struggling emotionally?
- What area of premedical study do you recommend?
- What technology is available at your school?
- Are any scholarships and loans available at your school, and if so, which ones?
- How long will it take before I know if I am accepted?
- What do your students say are the best aspects of the school?
- If I am granted acceptance, does your school allow students to defer enrollment into a class at a later date?
- Do you have any school housing for singles and/or families?
- What loans are available for students at your institution?
- Are students required to live in on-campus housing for a required amount of time?
- What schools are available for my children?
- What clubs and support groups are available for my family?
- Is your institution a not-for-profit or a for-profit institution?
- Are textbooks, microscopes, etc. available on location from your school or do I have to provide them?
- How many graduates have received the M.D. degree from your school?
- Has your school ever had to shut down due to financial or other reasons?
- Have you undergone, or will you soon be, changing the curriculum?
- Is there additional science coursework that you would recommend I take?
- How is the grading system designed?
- What year did the first medical school class start at your institution?
- Has your institution moved locations recently? If so, why?
- What percent of the graduating class secured residency spots upon graduation?
- How many students have transferred out of your program over the last 3 years?
- How many students have dropped out of your institution over the last 3 years? For what reasons?
- What selection criteria does your school use to select students?

Chapter 5

INTERNATIONAL GRADUATES IN CANADA

Canada is host to many international medical graduates who practice medicine inside of Canada. In 2004, the country official addressed potential barriers to licensure and medical practice in the country. The Canadian Task Force was formed in 2005 and funded by the Government of Canada's Foreign Credentials Recognition Program. A National International Medical Graduate (IMG) database was founded in 2005 to track the capacity of IMG's in the country and to assist with recruitment of IMG's to practice medicine in Canada. This database has provided a detailed picture of IMG's across the country. Data is gathered from seven regional and provincial IMG centers; all seventeen Canadian medical schools; nine medical regulatory agencies; the Royal College of Physicians and Surgeons; the College of Family Physicians of Canada; the Medical Council of Canada; and the College of Medicine in Quebec.

As of 2015, over 18,000 of the 75,000 practicing physicians in Canada graduated from a medical school outside of Canada. In the Northwest Territories and in Quebec, over 10% of the practicing physicians are IMG's. Over one-third of all physicians in Newfoundland and Saskatchewan are international graduates. Canada has IMG pathways that are determined primarily from the level of medical education that a student has undergone so that students may enter the country to ultimately practice medicine in Canada.

Physicians who trained outside of Canada are referred to not only as international medical graduates (IMG's) but also as Canadian's studying abroad (CSA's) if they are Canadian citizens. Canadian citizens can seek education in any country, but historically the majority has chosen to study in the United States, Ireland, Australia, and the Caribbean. More students have gone to the Caribbean more than any other location. During the years of 2011-2014, over 3,100 Canadians will have obtained their medical doctorate degree in a country other than Canada. It is estimated that nearly 90% of the IMG's that are Canadian citizens or residents desire to return to Canada to practice medicine.

The CaRMS gathered data in 2010 that describes the general characteristics of Canadian's studying abroad (CSA's). For CSA's, they are generally older than students entering medical school in Canada. While 46% of medical students studying in Canada have an average age of 26-30, nearly 75% of medical students abroad have an average age of 26-30. It is presumed that the age difference is largely due to student's who reapply after not achieving initial selection in Canada. Nearly 75% of CSA's have applied to a Canadian medical school at least one time, and 37% had applied at least two or more times. Twenty percent have at least one parent who is a physician.

The first step for IMG's is to pass the Medical Council of Canada Evaluating Exam (MCCEE). This test is a computer-based exam that is designed to evaluate the overall medical knowledge that a medical school graduate should have obtained prior to entering a medical residency training program. The Canadian National IMG Database records note that 19,081 IMG's challenged the MCCEE from 2005-2012 of which 30% were Canadian citizens. Of those who passed the MCCEE during this time, 49% were born in Canada.

RESIDENCY MATCH DATA IN CANADA

The data and material presented in this chapter are intended for review by international and Canadian medical school graduates as they prepare for medical residency. Data presented has been obtained from International Medical School graduates unless otherwise specified. This data does NOT include Canadian or U.S. medical school graduates unless otherwise specified. Information in the section is taken directly from the Office of Research and Informative Services - The Associations of Faculties of Medicine of Canada and the Canadian Resident Matching Service publication entitled - *Canadian Students Studying Medicine Abroad.*

The total numbers of Canadian residency positions has increased since 1994 when only 1,307 positions were available. This number had fallen to 1,117 positions in 2002 but has increased steadily since to 2,847 positions as of 2014. For Canadian graduates, there is 1.0 applicant for every 1.05 position.

Statistically, Canadian medical graduates apply for Family Medicine positions at the highest rate (38.2%), followed by Internal Medicine (14.2%), with all other disciplines ranking at 6% or less. The first choice of the majority of applicant's is Family Medicine by far at 51.3%, with the nearest percentile thereafter at 11.4% for Internal Medicine. In Canada, dedicated IMG positions are offered by discipline. The greatest number is in Family Medicine with 180 positions which compromise 49.5% of all dedicated IMG positions. On average, male and female applicants from Canada and from international medical schools match into their discipline of choice at the same rate. A total of 154 Canadian students were unmatched after the first attempt in 2014, while 1,618 international medical students were unmatched during this period.

In 2014, 39 medical graduates from the United States applied for match in the Canadian healthcare system with 24 matching on the first attempt. For international medical graduates in 2014, 374 out of 1,992 applicants matched on their first attempt. Some Canadian graduates also apply through the National Residency Matching Program (NRMP) in the United States. In 2014, 24 Canadian students participated in the NRMP from six different Canadian medical schools. Of these, only two Canadian students were successful in the match.

Table 5.1: 2014 Canadian Residency Match Results

Applicants	Matched	Unmatched
Canadian Medical Graduates	2779	123
International Medical Graduates	449	1869
U.S. Medical Graduates	27	14
Total	3255	2006

Source: Canadian Students Studying Medicine Abroad. Canadian Resident Matching Service

The Canadian medical education system uses the terms first and second iteration when discussing the match results. The first iteration refers to the first round in the residency match process and the second iteration refers to the second round of matching for students who were not successful in the first round. The following tables describe this information as it pertains to each medical school that offers residency programs.

Table 5.2: 2014 First Year Match Positions by Second Iteration

Location	Available Positions		Filled Positions		Unfilled Positions	
	1st Iteration	2nd Iteration	1st Iteration	2nd iteration	1st iteration	2nd Iteration
Dalhousie University	127	12	115	12	12	0
McGill University	182	4	178	1	4	3
McMaster University	222	15	207	14	15	1
Memorial University of Newfoundland	79	23	56	20	23	3
Northern Ontario School of Medicine	56	5	51	5	5	0
Queen's University	133	6	127	6	6	0
Universite de Montreal	228	23	265	10	23	13
Univerisite de Sherbrooke	199	24	175	13	24	11
Universite Laval	236	27	209	14	27	13
University of Alberta	204	18	186	9	18	9
University of British Columbia	328	10	318	7	10	3
University of Calgary	203	5	198	7	5	3
University of Manitoba	138	21	117	19	21	2
University of Ottawa	202	15	187	11	15	4
University of Saskatchewan	117	11	106	11	11	0
Western University	187	9	178	9	9	0
Total	3319	228	3091	164	228	64

Source: Canadian Students Studying Medicine Abroad. Canadian Resident Matching Service

Table 5.3: International Medical Graduates by Country - All Years of Training – 2013

Rank	Country MD Earned	Legal Status		Total	Language of Training in Canada	
		Canadian Citizens or Permanent Resident	Visa		English	French
1	Saudi Arabia	32	676	708	690	18
2	Ireland	277	77	354	353	1
3	India	126	168	294	294	0
4	Australia	140	100	240	240	0
5	Iran	179	5	184	173	11
6	United Kingdom	88	87	175	175	0
7	U.S.	11	58	169	169	0
8	Egypt	121	22	143	133	10
9	Pakistan	86	23	109	109	0
10	Saba	94	0	94	94	0
11	Israel	16	67	83	83	0
12	Grenada	75	0	75	75	0
13	China	49	22	71	71	0
13	Oman	0	71	71	71	0
15	Brazil	25	44	69	62	7
16	Poland	62	5	67	67	0
17	Saint Kitts and Nevis	59	0	59	59	0
18	Romania	54	3	57	43	14
19	Columbia	40	16	56	47	9
20	Japan	1	51	52	52	0
	119 others countries with less than 50 students					
Total		2348	2083	4431	4213	218

Source: Office of Research and Informative Services. The Associations of Faculties of Medicine of Canada

Table 5.4: Number of International Residency Positions by Location

Location	Number of Positions	Number of Matched IMG's
Dalhousie University	9	9
McGill University	N/A	18
McMaster university	34	32
Memorial University of Newfoundland	3	3
Northern Ontario School of Medicine	3	3
Queen's University	19	19
Universite de Montreal	N/A	7
Univerisite de Sherbrooke	N/A	7
Universite Laval	N/A	11
University of Alberta	19	16
University of British Columbia	42	41
University of Calgary	21	20
University of Manitoba	18	17
University of Ottawa	37	34
University of Saskatchewan	11	28
Western University	42	38
Total	329	374

Source: Canadian Students Studying Medicine Abroad. Canadian Resident Matching Service

Table 5.5: Number of Residency Positions Based on Location and Specialty

Residency Location	Family Medicine Positions	Royal College Positions	Total
Dalhousie University	59	68	127
McGill University	87	95	182
McMaster University	100	122	222
Memorial University of Newfoundland	33	46	78
Northern Ontario School of Medicine	37	19	56
Queen's University	68	64	133
Universite de Montreal	144	144	288
Univerisite de Sherbrooke	102	97	199
Universite Laval	117	119	236
University of Alberta	81	123	204
University of British Columbia	156	172	328
University of Calgary	92	111	203
University of Manitoba	56	82	136
University of Ottawa	70	132	202
University of Saskatchewan	45	72	117
Western University	77	110	187
Total	1487	1832	3319

Source: Canadian Students Studying Medicine Abroad. Canadian Resident Matching Service

Table 5.6: Match Applicants Per Discipline

Discipline	Number of Applicants – Canadian	Number of Applicants - International
Anatomical Pathology	43	164
Anesthesiology	202	204
Cardiac Surgery	18	36
Dermatology	84	67
Emergency Medicine	133	170
Family Medicine	1913	253
General Pathology	9	2206
General Surgery	183	122
Hematological Pathology	9	236
Internal Medicine	807	5
Laboratory Medicine	807	1072
Medical Biochemistry	4	126
Medical Genetics	10	15
Medical Microbiology	20	63
Neurology	79	18
Neurology – Pediatric	25	177
Neuropathology	1	56
Neurosurgery	23	55
Nuclear Medicine	24	3
OB / GYN	178	142
Ophthalmology	68	46
Orthopedic Surgery	89	145
Otolaryngology	44	4
Pediatrics	308	398
Physical Medicine and Rehab	46	126
Plastic Surgery	73	64
Psychiatry	260	497
Public Health/Preventive Med	30	206
Radiation Oncology	30	63
Urology	53	70
Vascular Surgery	19	63
Total	5018	6870

Source: Canadian Students Studying Medicine Abroad. Canadian Resident Matching Service

Table 5.7: IMG Dedicated Canadian Residency Positions

Discipline	Number of Dedicated Positions	Number of Positions	Number Filled	Number Vacant
Anatomical Pathology	1.8%	6	4	3
Anesthesiology	3.0%	11	10	1
Cardiac Surgery	0.3%	1	0	1
Dermatology	0.3%	1	1	0
Emergency Medicine	1.8%	6	6	0
Family Medicine	49.5%	180	176	4
General Pathology	0.6%	2	2	0
General Surgery	1.8%	6	6	0
Hematological Pathology	0.3%	1	0	1
Internal Medicine	15.2%	52	51	1
Laboratory Medicine	0.9%	4	4	0
Medical Genetics	0.3%	1	1	0
Medical Microbiology	0.3%	1	1	0
Neurology	1.5%	5	5	0
Neurology – Pediatric	0.3%	1	1	0
Neurosurgery	0.9%	3	2	1
OB / GYN	0.9%	3	3	0
Ophthalmology	0.3%	0	0	0
Orthopedic Surgery	1.8%	6	6	0
Pediatrics	5.8%	19	18	1
Physical Medicine and Rehab	1.2%	3	3	0
Plastic Surgery	0.3%	0	0	0
Psychiatry	7.0%	23	22	1
Public Health and Preventive Medicine	0.6%	2	1	1
Radiation Oncology	0.3%	1	1	0
Urology	0.9%	3	2	1
Vascular Surgery	0.3%	1	1	0
Total	346	100%	331	15

Source: Canadian Students Studying Medicine Abroad. Canadian Resident Matching Service

Table 5.8: Number of International Medical Graduate's by Graduation Region

Region	Numbers Attempting to Match	Number Matched	Percent Matched
Africa	358	40	11
Asia	462	35	8
Caribbean / Central America	528	131	25
Europe	478	146	31
Middle East	333	36	11
North America	9	3	33
Pacific Islands / Oceania	81	42	52
South America	69	16	23
Total	2318	449	19

Source: Canadian Students Studying Medicine Abroad. Canadian Resident Matching Service

It is very important to know how many residency spots are available for each specialty in Canada. This can be of particular interest to international medical school graduates as the availability of specific residencies may limit a student's choice of specialty options. This area should be carefully explored when planning the area of medicine in which the student wants to practice. Many international applicants apply to more than one specially. For example, a student interested in Pediatrics may also want to consider Family Medicine as a choice of specialty in order to obtain a match. The average hours that are worked during residency and the time spent on call are important to many when selecting a residency specialty.

Table 5.9: 2014 Match Results by Number and Discipline for Canadian and International Medical Graduates

Discipline	Canadian Medical Graduates	International Medical Graduates
Anatomical Pathology	22	7
Anesthesiology	104	10
Cardiac Surgery	7	1
Dermatology	31	1
Diagnostic Radiology	75	5
Emergency Medicine	69	7
Family Medicine	1184	203
General Pathology	4	2
General Surgery	86	7
Hematological Pathology	3	0
Internal Medicine	423	53
Laboratory Medicine	2	4
Medical Genetics	5	1
Medical Microbiology	7	1
Neurology	37	1
Neurology – Pediatric	6	1
Neurosurgery	14	3
Nuclear Medicine	7	0
OB / GYN	92	3
Ophthalmology	39	0
Orthopedic Surgery	54	6
Otolaryngology	28	0
Pediatrics	135	19
Physical Medicine and Rehab	23	3
Plastic Surgery	26	0
Psychiatry	143	24
Public Health and Preventive Medicine	9	4
Radiation Oncology	18	1
Urology	31	2
Vascular Surgery	9	1
Total	2693	374

Source: Canadian Students Studying Medicine Abroad. Canadian Resident Matching Service

Residency compensation will differ only slightly depending upon which field is chosen. Medical residents in Canada are compensated at a rate above the Canadian national wage index. The average Canadian first year salary is $49,000 CAD before taxes with first year residents receiving an average salary of $51,600 CAD. In general, not considering the cost of living, residents are compensated the most in Alberta, Manitoba, and Saskatchewan; at the average range in Newfoundland and Labrador, the Maritime Provinces, and Ontario; and the least in Quebec and British Columbia. The average compensation increases on average by 1-2% each year.

Table 5.10: Average Gross Annual Canadian Residency Compensation**

Medical School	PGY-1	PGY-2	PGY-3	PGY-4	PGY-5	PGY-6	PGY-7	PGY-8
Newfoundland and Labrador #	$53,282	$62,126	$66,339	$70,734	$75,495	$80,589	$83,325	No Data
Maritime Provinces*	$51,546	$60,102	$64,178	$68,429	$73,035	$77,963	$80,610	$86,252
Quebec^	$41,874	$45,951	$50,672	$54,370	$ 59,129	$62,098	$65,205	$68,463
Ontario^	$51,065	$59,608	$63,230	$67,512	$71,995	$76,210	$79,220	$83,704
Manitoba+	$54,956	$61,604	$66,080	$71,163	$76,247	$81,332	$86,314	$93,055
Saskatchewan*	$54,715	$59,671	$64,622	$69,552	$74,446	$79,328	No Data	No Data
Alberta#	$55,073	$61,066	$65,849	$70,637	$76,624	$81,411	$88,037	$95,207
British Columbia#	$49,934	$55,705	$60,702	$65,341	$70,268	$75,022	No Data	No Data

Source: Canadian Resident Matching Service   ^last updated in 2011 *last updated in 2012 #last updated in 2013 +last updated in 2014

** All funds are reported in Canadian funds

Chapter 6

Financial Aid

The cost of a Canadian medical education can be high. The overall cost of the education alone can go as high as $200,000 CAD in total tuition costs. The amount of the actual tuition can vary tremendously depending on the school, the geographic location of the applicant, and other variables. For international medical school applicants the cost of tuition is the highest. This is due to the fact that Canadian citizens, visa holders, landed immigrants, and in-province residents are charged much less with the cost often under-written, at least partially, by governmental agencies. The overall cost of the education is higher for both groups than just the actual tuition costs. Additional costs include travel, living expenses, fees, books, and other expenses. Each school will want to have proof that a student is able to pay for or finance their education prior to matriculation. Financial aid and scholarships can help to defer some of these expenses but are not guaranteed.

Many academic medical centers in Canada and the United States are having difficulty maintaining a cap on the current tuition charged to students. Despite the high cost of a medical education, the amount charged to the students does not cover the actual cost of the education. Many of these academic centers have historically made up the cost difference through hospital based education and research, but the demand for payment reform, and the shift of many areas of patient care into the outpatient setting has stressed the system. This decrease in revenue will have effects in the cost of training, or the processes used to offset these costs in the near future, but the actual way that this will occur is still unknown.

CANADIAN STUDENT LOAN PROGRAM

Student loans in Canada are designed to help post-secondary students pay for their education in Canada. The federal government funds the Canada Student Loan Program (CSLP) and the provinces may fund their own programs that run in parallel with the federal CSLP. In addition, most Canadian banks offer commercial loans targeted for students in medical education programs. Canadian citizens and permanent residents of Canada are those that live in any province for over a year, and they are normally eligible for loans provided by the federal government through the CSLP.

Prior to 1964, the national student loan program was known as the Dominion-Provincial Student Loan Program. This program was a matching grant partnership system between the federal and provincial governments. This ended in 1964 when the CSLP started. Since the inception of CSLP, the program has supplemented the financial resources available to eligible students from other sources to assist in their pursuit of post-secondary education. Between 1964 and 1995, loans were provided by financial institutions to post-secondary students who were approved to receive financial assistance. The financial institutions also administered the loan repayment process. In return, the Government of Canada guaranteed each Canadian Student Loan that was issued by reimbursing the financial institution the full amount of any loans that went into default.

Several important changes were made to the program in 1995. First, the Canada Student Financial Assistance Act was initiated replacing the existing Canada Student Loans Act reflecting the changing needs of the parties involved in the loan process including the banks. The Government of Canada developed a formalized "risk-shared" agreement with several financial institutions, with the institution assuming responsibility for the possible risk of defaulted loans in return for a fixed payment from the Government.

The risk-shared arrangement between the Government of Canada and participating financial institutions came to an end in 2000. The Government of Canada now directly finances all new loans issued on or after August 1, 2000. The administration of Canada Student Loans program has become the responsibility of the National Student Loans Service Centre (NSLSC). There are two divisions of the NSLSC. One manages loans for students attending public institutions and the other administers loans for students attending private institutions.

Due to the close nature of the CSLP and the provincial student loan programs, the changes in 1995 and 2000 were largely mirrored by the provincial programs. As a result of these changes, students who attended school before and after these transition years found that they had up to six different loans to manage. The extent to which this is possible depends largely on a student's province of residence. Currently, the loans issued to full-time students are interest free while a student is engaged in full-time studies. Students receiving a Canada Student Loan (CSL) are eligible for up to 340 weeks (~6.5 years) of interest-free assistance while obtaining their education. Students in doctoral programs are eligible for an additional 60 weeks for up to 400 weeks (~7.5 years).

As the length of Canadian graduate degree programs often exceeds this 400 week maximum, students considering graduate study are advised to think carefully before taking out student loans. Graduate students can easily find themselves in a position where they no longer qualify for student loans. Students in full-time study are not required to repay their student loans while still in their course of study even if they have exceeded the length of time that loans are available.; however, interest begins to accumulate immediately upon reaching the lifetime limit.

Students must apply for the Canadian and provincial loans through their provincial government. The rules for what determines the province of residence vary, but normally it is defined as the geographical location where a student has most recently lived for at least 12 consecutive months, not including time spent as a full-time student at a post-secondary institution. In most cases, the province of residence is the province one lived in before becoming a post-secondary student.

Canada Student Loans offer up to $210 CAD per week for full-time study or 60% of the student's assessed need (the lesser of these) can be issued per loan year (August 1–July 31). Loans issued through provincial programs will normally provide students with enough funding to cover the balance of their assessed need.

Determining Your Eligibility

To be eligible for a Canada Student Loan, for full-time studies, a student must satisfy all of the following:

- Be a Canadian citizen, a permanent resident of Canada, or a protected person (including convention refugees);
- Be a resident of a territory or province that issues Canada Student Loans;
- Demonstrate financial need;
- Be enrolled in minimum 60 percent of a full course load (students with permanent disabilities may enroll in a minimum 40 percent of a full course load);
- Be enrolled in a degree, diploma, or certificate program of at least 12 weeks in length (within a period of 15 consecutive weeks) at a designated educational institution;
- Maintain a satisfactory scholastic standard; and
- Pass a credit check if 22 years of age or older and applying for a Canada Student Loan for the first time.

For each program of study, students are eligible for student loans for the number of periods of study it normally takes to complete that program plus one period.

The salaries of physicians depend upon a number of factors to include the specialty, experience, and the geographical location within the country where the physician practices. A prospective student should keep in mind that regardless of the study or article that they may read on physician salaries that salaries change rapidly in today's healthcare environment. All students should become informed and be realistic about how much money they can earn when they graduate. Students need to identify their income range for at least five years. The income that can be earned during the internship and residency is also important. Once the income is identified, the student should take the gross income and reduce it by twenty-five to thirty percent to account for federal, state/provincial, and other taxes. The amount left over is what will be left for repayment of the student loans and for living expenses.

When making payments, it is helpful to write checks rather than to use money orders if at all possible when dealing with each school. By doing this, it will be possible to know when the school has processed the application from the date that the check was processed. This will also provide a reliable method of tracking monies received by the various institutions.

HOW MUCH FINANCIAL AID TO ACCEPT

When deciding how much financial aid that a student wants to apply for, many factors must be considered. To begin, students should review all sources of financial support to include parental support, support from relatives, and support from friends. For married students, spousal income will be a major source of support. Students should also seek grants or scholarships through companies or corporations, fraternal organizations, and religious groups. The average debt for medical school graduates in the United States and Canada is $167,750 CAD.

The two main sources for financing medical school are loans and grants. Loans must be repaid and have varying interests rates, while grants do not have to be paid back but may have associated stipulations such as requiring work in a certain location for a certain period of time after residency training. Grants will often have specific stipulations as well based on citizenship, gender, associations, and other variables.

Students must review their current debts. If student loans have already been taken, can the payments be deferred? If so, will interest be charged while the student is in school? Does the student have a car payment, a mortgage, or credit card debt? Can these balances be reduced or paid off before starting school? Any debt that can be reduced or removed prior to beginning medical school is a plus.

Canadian students should also review their credit rating. Look at the rating before, not after, enrollment. Students will have a difficult time obtaining student loans if they have ever had a bankruptcy, defaulted on a student loan, or had a tax lien or a civil judgment entered against them. Many lenders will refuse to grant student loans if the student habitually pays their accounts slowly. The credit reporting agencies will charge a fee to obtain a credit report although some companies may allow one free copy each year. Anyone who has been denied credit in the last 60 days is entitled to a free credit report.

The credit criteria used to approve student loans will include the following:

- Absence of negative credit

- No bankruptcies, repossessions, foreclosures, open judgments, or charge-offs

- No prior educational loan defaults unless paid in full or making satisfactory progress in repayment

- Absence of excessive past due accounts

- No 30, 60 or 90-day delinquencies on consumer loans or revolving charge accounts within the past two years.

Canada has two national credit bureaus: Equifax Canada and TransUnion Canada. Both of these organizations operate in the United States as well. The United States has a third credit agency, Experian, as well. Students are able to check with both bureaus and receive a free copy of their credit file.

Table 6.1: Canadian Credit Reporting Agencies

NAME	ADDRESS	TELEPHONE
EQUIFAX (http://www.consumer.equifax.ca/)	Equifax Canada Co. Box 190 Jean Talon Station Montreal, Quebec H1S 2Z2	1-800-465-7166
TRANS UNION CORPORATION (https://www.transunion.ca/ca)	**For English correspondence:** TransUnion Attention: Consumer Relations P.O. Box 338, LCD1 Hamilton, ON L8L 7W2 **For French correspondence:** TransUnion Centre de relations au consommateur CP 1433 Succ. St-Martin Laval, QC H7V 3P7	**For English correspondence:** 1-800-663-9980 **For French correspondence:** 1-877-713-3393 514-335-0374 in Montreal

Table 6.2 Financial Aid Rights and Responsibilities

Financial Aid Rights
• The right to examine your financial aid information at any time
• The right to accept or decline all or part of the aid offered
• The right to expect assistance from the Financial Aid Office
• The right that your financial information is private
• The right to appeal your financial aid package if your financial situation changes
• The right not to be discriminated against based of age, race, creed, gender, handicap, or national origin
Financial Aid Responsibilities
• To read and understand the terms and conditions of the financial aid package
• To meet the expense related to the medical school educations
• To submit financial aid applications on time
• To report any outside funding, including scholarships and loans, that you are receiving
• To obtain and complete financial aid forms supplying the necessary and relevant information
• To use loan funds to pay tuition
• To notify lenders of any changes of address
• To keep accurate and complete records of all financial aid applications and transactions
• To repay all loans

Source: The Best 167 Medical Schools, 2015 Edition. The Princeton Review

BUDGETING

Students must plan a realistic expense budget. Many schools provide budgets for their students but these should be regarded as guidelines only. Students will have different lifestyles, needs, and wants; and the finances required by individual students can vary greatly.

Table 6.3: Monthly Student Budget

LIVING EXPENSES	ACTUAL - 20____	PROJECTED - 20____
Rent/mortgage/housing		
Utilities: Gas/oil		
Electricity		
Water		
Telephone		
Groceries: Food		
Household supplies		
Transportation: subway/bus		
Gasoline		
Car Maintenance		
Other:_____		
Savings		
Credit Cards		
Insurance: Health		
Life		
Auto		
Entertainment: Meals out		
Movies/concerts/theater		
Health club, etc.		
Personal: clothes/laundry		
Grooming(e.g. haircuts)		
Other:_____		
Miscellaneous:		

MONTHLY LIVING BUDGET		
1st and 2nd year students multiply the BUDGET by 9*; **3rd and 4th year students multiply the budget by 12.**		

Original Source: Philadelphia College of Osteopathic Medicine

Table 6.4: Yearly Student Budget

EDUCATIONAL EXPENSES	ACTUAL - 20____	PROJECTED - 20____
Tuition		
Fees		
Books		
Supplies		
Special Equipment		
Other:_____		
TOTAL EDUCATIONAL EXPENSES:		
TOTAL LIVING EXPENSES:		
TOTAL LIVING AND EDUCATIONAL EXPENSES:		
INCOME/RESOURCES:		
Money from: Savings:		
Parents/Spouse:		
Work-Study:		
Other Work:		
Scholarships/Grants:		
Loans: Stafford Subsidized:		
Stafford unsubsidized:		
Federal Perkins Loan:		
Primary Care Loan:		
Alternative Loan:		

TOTAL INCOME/RESOURCES:		
INCOME (minus) EXPENSES:		

Original Source: Philadelphia College of Osteopathic Medicine

The amount of loans taken out should be tied to potential income that the physician will make in the future. A good "rule-of-thumb" is that the total amount of student loans should not be greater than the income of the first year of practice. The table below provides some guidance based on average physician salaries. The salaries are an average, and significant variation in physician salaries depends on the region, location, market demand, and other factors.

Table 6.5: Physician Compensation

Medical Specialty	Annual Income (CAD)
Anesthesiology	$405,000
General / Family Practice	$210,000
Internal Medicine	$222,000
OB/GYN	$291,000
Pathology	$297,000
Pediatrics	$208,000
Psychiatry	$224,000
Radiation Therapy	$419,000
Surgery	$335,000

Source: The Princeton Review. The Best 167 Medical Schools, 2015 Edition

LOANS

Many schools offer supplemental loans which may provide for some or all of the funds needed to attend medical school. Institutional loans are offered at terms and conditions that generally have higher interest rates and fees than government sponsored loans. Eligibility requirements, terms and conditions, and credit criteria vary with different programs and can frequently change.

Every bank will charge a fee when a student obtains a student loan. The fee covers an origination fee and a guarantee fee. The bank retains the origination fee and the guarantee fee is sent to the agency that guarantees or insures the loan. Because banks compete for business, they will rarely charge the maximum fees allowed by law. An example is if $20,000 is borrowed with a 3% fee, the student will receive $19,400. If $20,000 is borrowed with a 7% fee, the student will receive $18,600. When repayment begins, the principal is what is repaid, not the net. Interest is also computed on the principal and not the net.

Repayment on the student loans will begin after residency is completed and after the grace period has expired. Most repayment terms will span 10, 20, or even 30 years. Longer repayment terms will result in the student paying more interest. Many private loans are available from multiple sources. The most common and utilized resources are described below.

ADDITIONAL FINANCIAL SOURCES

Canada Student Grants Program: This program combines all federal grants into one plan. Applicants must apply for a grant and demonstrate financial need. If the application is accepted, students may be eligible for grant money which does not have to be repaid upon graduation. Grants are also available for individuals who fall into certain categories, such as those who are disabled or are supporting children while attending school.

International Professions Education Loan Program (TERI) - Provides $18,000 CAD per academic year. The loan is non-need based and requires a co-signer and/or a co-borrower. It is available to U.S. citizens or permanent residents but can also be received by Canadian residents who can provide a credit-worthy U.S. co-signer.

Veterans Benefits - Dependent upon each individual case. Veterans should contact the Canadian Department of Veterans' Affairs.

International Select Alternative Loan - Provides up to $35,000 USD per year for U.S. students and $24,000 CAD for two semesters of full-time study for Canadian residents. This loan is designed to cover the difference between the attendance cost and the amount that other loans provide. This loan is available to U.S. citizens or permanent residents and Canadian students with good credit histories. The Educational Finance Group (EFG) administers this loan.

Professional Edge Student Program – Offered by the Canadian Imperial Bank of Commerce and allows students access to funds while attending an accredited Canadian university or college and for 12 months after graduation or residency. Applicants pay interest only while in school or residency and can take up to $275,000 CAD in total.

Key Education Loan - Key Education Resources provides products and services through the Key Bank in the United States. Loans are available from Key Education Resources to include the MedAchiever loan and the MedAchiever Residency Travel and Relocation loan. The Key Alternative loan and the Alternative DEAL's Best BET (Board Exam and Travel) loans are also available.

MedAchiever Loan - Provides annually up to the cost of education minus other forms of financial aid. The minimum loan amount is $600 CAD and no payments are required during school and for the 48 months after graduation. This loan is offered through the Key Bank, USA and is available for U.S. citizens and permanent residents only.

ED-Invest Foreign Medical School Student Loan Program – Designed for international medical school programs and students. This program provides funding in variable amounts and at varying interest rates for select applicants.

Loan Forgiveness - A Canadian Student Loan forgiveness program for physicians is available for the purpose of expanding the provision of primary health services. The program is designed to encourage and support new family physicians to practice in underserved rural or remote communities of the country including communities that provide health services to First Nation and the Inuit populations.

Provincial and Territorial School Loans

Once a student maximizes federal benefits or has been denied federal financial assistance, they may be able to find support from the Canadian province or territory where they reside.

Alberta: The Alberta Learning Information Service offers scholarships, bursaries, and school loans. Financial planning resources are also available.

British Columbia: StudentAidBC provides loans, scholarships, grants, and other services. They also have special information for applicants who have dependents, disabilities, use income assistance, or have other unique situations.

Manitoba: Students can apply for tuition loans and grants through Manitoba Student Aid. Medical students are eligible for additional medical grants.

New Brunswick: Applicants can apply for full-time or part-time student assistance through New Brunswick's Student Financial Services.

Newfoundland and Labrador: Financial assistance options are available via Newfoundland and Labrador Student Aid. Additional grant and aid options are available as well.

Northwest Territories: Student handbooks, policies, procedures, and applications for aid are available from NWT Student Financial Assistance.

Nova Scotia: The Nova Scotia Student Assistance department has several student aid options. Students can apply for student loans and receive assistance in finding approved institutions.

Ontario: The Ontario Student Assistance Program seeks to provide financial support to its residents through student loans, grants, scholarships, and bursaries.

Prince Edward Island: Students may apply for provincial loans through PEI Student Financial Services.

Quebec: Loans and bursaries are available for both full-time and part-time students from the Aide financier aux etudes.

Saskatchewan: Student loan options are available through the Saskatchewan Student Financial Assistance program.

Yukon Territory: Student aid is available from Yukon Student Financial Assistance. Grants, loans, scholarships, awards, and other funds are available.

Chapter 7

Licensure

The steps to becoming a licensed physician in Canada have different starting points for those trained in Canada and those trained internationally This can be confusing to applicants in training, particularly for students trained outside of Canada. Variations in the licensure requirements across Canada add to the confusion as does variation in provincial requirements.

The required steps to become licensed in Canada are as follows:

Step 1: Medical Council of Canada Evaluating Examination (MCCEE) – If not trained in Canada

Step 2: Medical Council of Canada Qualifying Examination (MCCQE) Part I – all applicants

Step 3: AMRCB® Certification (Currently Discretionary) – Primarily non-Canadian graduates

Step 4: National Assessment Collaboration (NAC) Examination – for some IMG's

Step 5: Completion of a Canadian (or United States) medical residency

Step 6: Medical Council of Canada Qualifying Examination (MCCQE) Part II
--or the --
Certification Examination in Family Medicine

To eventually become licensed as a practicing physician in Canada, international medical students first pass the Medical Council of Canada Evaluating Examination (MCCEE). This test is taken by international medical students and graduates and U.S. osteopathic physicians who desire to take the Medical Council of Canada Qualifying Examination (MCCQE) Part I and II. The Medical Council of Canada Qualifying Examination (MCCQE) Part I must be taken by all applicants. Applicants must first have passed the

MCCEE or have trained in Canada. The MCCQE is designed to assess the overall competence of candidates who have obtained a medical degree. The MCCQE Part II is taken by all candidates who have passed the MCCQE Part I, and is designed to assess the overall knowledge, attitudes, and skills needed to qualify for an independent medical license in Canada. All 12 licensing authorities in Canada require the passing of the MCCQE Steps I and either the MCCQE Step II or the Certification Examination in Family Medicine to practice independently. The National Assessment Collaboration (NAC) Examination is required in some regions for eligibility for postgraduate residency training which is required for eventual independent practice of medicine in Canada.

American Medical Residency Certification Board (AMRCB®) completion is utilized by international graduates to demonstrate a sign of excellence and to access readiness to enter a U.S. or Canadian medical internship or residency position. AMRCB® certification remains voluntary at the time of this publication. AMRCB® certification evaluates, trains, and ranks international medical students and graduates on professionalism; presentations skills; the ability to apply information and knowledge; attention to detail; communication skills; motivation; organization; and the ability to relate to people. AMRCB® certification can be achieved at any time during the medical education process. The majority of students take the course during their third and fourth year clinical rotations as they are applying to U.S. and Canadian residency positions although many others choose to take the course early on during their educational journey.

Medical students and graduates are encouraged to contact the medical regulatory authority in the province or territory they are considering practicing in. Many territories and provinces have an international medical graduate program as well that can provide additional guidance. International medical graduates must also have graduated from a recognized medical school. A recognized medical school is one that is listed by the International Medical Education Directory (IMED). IMED is part of the Foundation for Advancement of International Medical Education and Research (FAIMER). Recognized medical schools can be located on the FAIMER website at: http://www.faimer.org/resources/imed.html.

MEDICAL COUNCIL OF CANADA EVALUATIONING EXAMINATION (MCCEE)

The MCCEE is designed to test a student's general knowledge on the principles of medicine. The principles include Community Health, Internal Medicine, Obstetrics/Gynecology, Pediatrics, Preventive Medicine, Psychiatry, and Surgery. The examination is a four hour, computer-based examination that consists of 180 multiple choice questions, each which lists five possible answers with only one correct answer. The MCCEE is offered in both French and English. The MCCEE is currently offered at more than 500 centers in over 80 countries. International medical students and graduates and U.S. osteopathic medical students are eligible to take the examination during the final 20 months of their medical education. The MCCEE is a prerequisite for eligibility to take the Medical Council of Canada Qualifying examinations for international graduates.

Each question is designed to test a specific patient group and clinical task. Five specific Patient Groups are used and include: Adult Health; Child Health; Maternal Health; Mental Health; and Population Health and Ethics. Three Clinical Tasks are used and include: Data Gathering; Data Interpretation and Synthesis; and Management. The overall purpose of the MCCEE is to assess the knowledge and skills required at the level of a new medical graduate who is entering into supervised resident training.

Scoring on the MCCEE is based upon a student's overall score in relation to the cutoff passing score which is currently set at 250. Grading does not follow a curve where a predetermined number of students pass, fail, or fall into certain percentile categories. The MCCEE is not designed to be a barrier for examinees to prevent them from entering the path for the MCC Qualifying Examination for Canadian licensure; therefore, scoring is less difficult than for the MCCQE Part I. Passing the MCCEE does not guarantee passing on the MCCQE. The goal of scoring on the MCCEE is to allow students to demonstrate the minimum competence needed to pursue additional medical education in the Canadian system. Scores become available on the physiciansapply.ca account which is set up prior to taking the test. Information is provided which helps the applicant interpret their scores in total and by individual disciplines, patient groups, and clinical tasks. No limit exists as to the number of times that an applicant may take the test, although once a student passes the test, they may not take the test again for any reason (for example, to obtain a higher score). Results from the MCC examination are released approximately seven weeks after the last day of the examination period.

The MCCEE is given in multiple locations in Canada and in international locations as well. Applications for the test are accepted throughout the year. The scheduling for particular examinations closes 120 hours prior to the examination date and time. The examination is given several times each year in block periods ranging from 10 days to three weeks. Questions on the MCCEE are based on objectives that are published by the MCC each year in a document entitled *Objectives for the Qualifying Examination*. The current cost of the test is $1,645 CAD.

Table 7-1: Description of MCCEE Patient Groups and Clinical Tasks

Patient Groups	Clinical Tasks
Adult Health Issues particular to individuals after the end of adolescence	Data Gathering History taking, mental status examination, physical examination, laboratory testing, and other modalities (imaging, EKG, EEG, etc.)
Child Health Issues particular to individuals up to the end of adolescence	Data Interpretation and Synthesis Interpretation and synthesis of gathered data. Problem identification, setting priorities, and risk stratification. Formulation of differential and specific diagnosis.
Maternal Health Issues related to pregnancy and childbirth	Management Education and health promotion, counseling, psychotherapy, drug and non-drug therapy (includes fluid and electrolyte therapy), surgical interventions, radiological interventions, cessation of therapy, rehabilitation, palliative care, interdisciplinary management, and family and community care.
Mental Health Biopsychosocial/cognitive issues related to mental health in all age groups	
Population Health and Ethics Issues related to groups and ethical behavior. Includes population issues such as disease outbreak management; epidemiology and relevant statistics; health promotion strategies; immunization; and population screening and surveillance. Ethical issues include boundary issues, impairment of doctors, and informed consent.	

MCCEE Self-Administered Evaluating Examinations (SAE-EE and SAE-QEI)

International Medical Graduates are able to assess their readiness to take the MCCEE and the MCCQE Step I by taking practice examinations. Applicants can take the Self-Administered Evaluation Examination (SAE-EE) and the Self-Administered Qualifying Examination Part I (SAE-QEI). The Self-Administered

Examinations are internet-based and consist of 96 questions from six different medical disciplines. The tests are available 24 hours a day, and students are allowed four hours over a seven-day period to complete the test. The majority of students complete the examination over 2.5 hours. Upon completion, students receive feedback by e-mail which provides the number of correct answers and a comparison of results to others who have taken the test. The SAE examinations do not cover all of the material that is covered on the MCCEE or the MCCQE Part I. The SAE examinations are not meant to take the place of other examinations and are provided as a study aid as students prepare to take the formal examinations. The results are not stored, and the tests are meant for use by the participants only. IMG's must create an account and submit all materials to the MCC Physician Credential Repository prior to becoming eligible for the MCCEE. The MCCEE is necessary to enter the Canadian Resident Matching service.

The Self-Administered Evaluation Examination (SAE-EE) is a series of multiple choice practice examinations. The test is designed to assess the level of preparedness of medical school graduates to take the MCCEE. Candidates who take this test receive the number of questions that they correctly answered and their percentile to compare their performance with others taking the test. The medical disciplines include Medicine, OB/GYN, Pediatrics, Psychiatry, and Surgery. The SAE-EE includes a sixth discipline which includes ommunity health and preventive medicine questions.

The Self-Administered Qualifying Examination Part I (SAE-QEI) is designed to assess the readiness of applicants to take the MCCQE Part I. The medical disciplines include Medicine, OB/GYN, Pediatrics, Psychiatry, and Surgery. The SAE-QEI includes a sixth discipline which includes questions on the ethical, legal, and organizational aspects of medicine as well as questions on population health. Unlike the MCCQE Part I, the SAE-QEI does not contain questions on clinical decision making, although clinical decision making content is expected to be added in the future. As such, the SAE-QEI can only be used for preparation for the MCCQE Part I.

MEDICAL COUNCIL OF CANADA QUALIFYING EXAMINATION (MCCQE)

The MCCQE Parts I and II are designed based on educational objectives. The objectives are designed to reflect the necessary knowledge of competent physicians. Both tests operate on the assumption that it is better to prevent disease than to treat it. Rational treatment decisions can only be made after an affective diagnosis has been established. The educational objectives deal with diagnostic and clinical problem solving, data gathering, and the principles of disease management. Questions are most often tied to clinical situations that are faced by practicing physicians.

MCCQE Step I

The MCCQE Part I is a multiple choice computer-based examination that tests basic medical knowledge similar to the MCCEE and USMLE®. The test is designed for applicants who have, or are near completion, of their medical degree. The MCCQE Part I is required prior to students being able to enter into supervised clinical practice in residency. The MCCQE Part I includes questions that are unique to physicians in Canada such as legal issues and include a half-day session on clinical decision making and clinical reasoning. The MCCQE Part I is only administered in Canada and the current cost of the examination is $920 CAD.

The MCCQE Part I is given in two sessions over one day. The first session is given in the morning over three and a half hours and students complete 196 multiple-choice questions. The second session is given over four hours in the afternoon and consists of short-menu and short-answer write-in questions that focus on clinical decision making.

The MCCQE Part I is scored independently from the MCCQE Part II. The MCCQE Part I is scored on a range of 50-950. A certain passing score is determined and students are not graded in comparison to how well others scored on the examination. Comparative information is included on the scoring report, however, for feedback purposes. The passing score is determine by MCC's Central Examination Committee (CEC) and is updated periodically. Prior to 2015, the passing score was 390 for Part I. The passing score for future tests is currently under review by the CEC. The passing score is determined by the CEC with input from faculty involved with training medical graduates across Canada. The final score is determined by calculating the combined scores from the clinical decision-making questions and the multiple-choice questions. For the clinical decision making questions, depending on the question and how many parts the question has, students receive a score of 0.25, 0.5, 0.75, or 1.0 per question. For multiple-choice questions, correct answers are assigned a value of 1.0 and incorrect answers are scored with a zero. Scores are verified a minimum of three times, and any borderline passing scores are given close scrutiny. Students can request to have the test re-scored.

Scores are released in June for the test given in the spring and in December for the test given in the fall. Candidates receive an e-mail notifying them that they can access their scores via their physiciansapply.ca account. No limit exists as to how many times a student can take the examination, although once a student has successfully passed the test, they no longer are eligible to take the test again for any reason.

MCCQE Part II

The MCCQE Part II is designed for applicants who have successfully completed the MCCQE Part I. This test is a three hour objective-structured clinical examination. The examination consists of questions covering community health and preventive medicine; general medicine and healthcare; Medicine; Pediatrics; OB/GYN; Psychiatry; Surgery; and other similar disciplines. The test is designed to assess the knowledge, attitudes, and skills necessary for independent medical practice in Canada. Family Medicine residents and College of Family Physicians of Canada (CFPC) practice eligible students are encouraged to the take the Certification Examination in Family Medicine instead of the MCCQE Part II. The MCCQE Part II is only administered in Canada and the current cost of the examination is $2,190 CAD. Candidates generally take the examination in the fall of their second year of residency training.

The MCCQE Part II consists of multiple clinical stations that contain common or critical patient presentations. The clinical stations contain a brief written statement that introduces a clinical problem. Applicants then interact with a standardized patient and perform a history and physical examination and are expected to address the issue and concerns of the patient. Candidates may be asked to interpret x-rays, make a diagnosis, write admission orders, answer specific questions, or to complete other medically related tasks. For each clinical station, students should identify the key diagnosis and the critical information required to diagnose and treat the condition. Pilot (non-scoring) stations are also often included to test the validity of future stations.

Scores are released by the MCC Central Examination Committee in June for the test given in the spring and in December for the test given in the fall. Candidates receive an e-mail notifying them that they can access their scores via their physiciansapply.ca account. The candidate's final score and the score required to pass the examination are displayed. Candidates also receive supplemental feedback. For candidates who pass the examination they will receive official licentiate documents by mail. No limit exists as to how many times a student can take the examination, although once a student successfully passes the examination; they no longer are eligible to take the test again for any reason. Students who do not pass the examination may request a re-score.

A new examination structure for Family Medicine physicians is now in place in Canada which is designed to increase the overall numbers of physicians across the country. With changes in the examination structure in 2015, demand is expected to be high for the MCCQE Part II examination. Family Medicine physicians are encouraged to take the Certification in Family Medicine Examination instead of the MCCQE Part II.

CERTIFICATION EXAMINATION IN FAMILY MEDICINE

The Certification Examination in Family Medicine was launched in 2013 by the Medical Council of Canada and the College of Family Physicians of Canada (CFPC). The purpose is to merge concepts from MCCQE Part II and the CFPC's Certification examination allowing students to only take one examination. All candidates must meet eligibility requirements for both the MCC and the CFPC, have successfully completed the MCCQE Part I, and have valid medical credentials. Candidates must have completed a CFPC-accredited family medicine program or have graduated from jurisdictions with similar standards of accreditation. Jurisdictions with similar standards of accreditation includes ACGME approved U.S. family medicine programs; AMC accredited Australian general practice vocational training programs; accredited general practice vocational training schemes of the Irish College of General Practitioners; and GMC accredited programs in the United Kingdom.

All candidates must be a registered member of the College of Family Physicians of Canada. Medical residents are eligible to take the examination during their last 6 months of training, regardless if the training program is 24 or 36 months in length. Practicing physicians are also eligible to take the examination and there are two eligibility tracks in place for those currently practicing medicine.

The examination consists of a clinical skills component and a written component. The clinical skills component consists of eight, 10-minute objective structured clinical examinations (OSCE's) and four, 15-minute simulated office oral examinations. The written component consists of multiple short answer management problems and is given over six hours. The short answer management problems are designed to evaluate the problem solving abilities, recall of factual knowledge, and critical appraisal needed to practice family medicine. Both the written and clinical skills components of the examination must be successfully completed.

The examination is offered in the spring and fall each year in multiple testing sites across Canada. Testing is available in French and English and candidates may take one component of the test in French and the other in English if desired. Testing sites in the spring are located in Calgary, Edmonton, Winnipeg, Hamilton, Toronto, Ottawa, Halifax, Kingston, London, Saskatoon, Vancouver, Montreal (French and English), Quebec (French), and Sherbrooke (French). Testing sites in the fall are located in Calgary, Toronto, Hamilton, Ottawa, and Montreal (French). The current cost of the examination is $4,845 CAD. Candidates who pass the examination are granted certification by the CFPC and Licentiate of the MCC.

AMERICAN MEDICAL RESIDENCY CERTIFICATION BOARD® (AMRCB®)

The American Medical Residency Certification Board (AMRCB®) was created to formalize the process of recognizing international excellence in medical education. The AMRCB® provides certification for international medical schools and for international medical students and graduates. The AMRCB® operates under the principle that many graduates of international medical institutions desire to practice medicine in a location other than the country where they attended medical school. The scope of the AMRCB® is to recognize the value of international medical training programs and their graduates within the United States and Canada.

The initial concept for the AMRCB® was conceived in the 1990's. A consortium was called of practicing physicians from the United States and the international community to establish and define the policies and procedures that would be necessary in order to appropriately understand the medical training that occurs across the globe. Through this effort, the official certification process for medical institutions and for medical students who desire to enter programs within the United States and Canada was begun in 2013.

For international medical students, it is not mandated that all have AMRCB® certification prior to entering a medical training program within the United States and Canada at this time. It is, however, being currently adopted by multiple agencies and organizations. The majority of students take the course during their third and fourth year clinical rotations as they are preparing to apply to residency positions. Many others choose to take the course early on during their educational journey. The course is not focused on specific medical topics, but on professionalism; presentation skills; the ability to apply information and knowledge; attention to detail; communication skills; motivation; organization; and the ability to relate to people. The AMRCB® emphasizes the concept that professional skills are the foundation of success not only in the field of medicine, but in every successful organization. AMRCB® certification will help international graduates who seek to be distinguished from the large pool of yearly applicants for internship and residency positions, and for those who want to achieve a mark of excellence.

AMRCB® student certification can be achieved at any time during the medical education process. It may be taken before, during, or after the MCCEE, MCCQE, USMLE® and ECFMG®(for U.S. applicants) testing requirements. The AMRCB® differs from the ECFMG® as the AMRCB® provides focused qualitative assessment and training that evaluates multiple different professional skills necessary for the practice of medicine in the U.S. and Canada. All applicants who undergo the certification process will not receive it, although the vast majorities who attend and complete the conference do receive certification. Course attendees receive a qualitative assessment and are ranked among those who have completed the course. A transcript of the educational scores and assessments are available to the student and are sent, upon request, to individual U.S., Canadian, and international medical residencies and other organizations as well.

TABLE 7.2: AMRCB® 2013-2014 Certification Pass Rates

	U.S. and Canadian Students	International Medical Students
AMRCB® First Attempt	95%	91%
AMRCB® Repeaters	98%	88%

Source: AMRCB® 2014 Data Report

NATIONAL ASSESSMENT COLLABORATION EXAMINATION (NAC)

The National Assessment Collaboration (NAC) Examination is required by some provinces in order to assess readiness for entering into a Canadian residency program. The NAC is an alliance of Canadian organizations that work to make the process of obtaining a license in Canada easier to obtain for International Medical Graduates. The NAC is only offered in Canada and is a national standardized examination. The examination is designed to test the skills, attitudes, and knowledge needed for postgraduate training in Canada. Students must have first taken and passed the MCCEE prior to becoming eligible to take the NAC examination although other criteria may apply in some jurisdictions. Students can take the test in any location, not just the province where they desire residency training.

The NAC asks questions on clinical scenarios based on a series of clinical stations. Medical questions include Gynecology, Medicine, Obstetrics, Pediatrics, Psychiatry, and Surgery. Candidates receive feedback on their results and on their weaknesses and strengths. Candidates are able to share the results of the test with residency programs if desired. As with the AMRCB® transcript, NAC results are accepted as part of the Canadian Resident Matching Service (CaRMS). The NAC is not, however, required to obtain a medical license in Canada, but may be required to be eligible for acceptance for residency training programs in some locations.

The NAC is currently offered in British Columbia, Calgary, Edmonton, Toronto, Vancouver, Halifax, Winnipeg, and Montreal. The cost is $2,230 CAD. Examination results are available within six to eight weeks after the completion of the examination.

TRANSFERRING TO THE UNITED STATES OR CANADA

The low attrition rate in the United States and Canada is by design. Students have worked extremely hard to obtain medical school positions and will do everything to avoid losing their place. Medical schools in the U.S. and Canada also work very hard to prevent students from failing out due to the public and private money that is invested in the education of each student. Spots will, however, still become available. Many U.S. and Canadian schools offer a remediation program for students having difficulty or for those who have failed classes. These students will often be allowed to repeat year one or year two and to continue their education. This results in openings for the clinical years while no students have actually left the program. The easiest schools to transfer into will be the schools who offer this opportunity for their students. This is still a difficult process and one that only a few students navigate successfully.

Although clearly the majority of students in Canada desire to train and eventually practice medicine in Canada, some may desire to study or practice medicine elsewhere. Some matriculate into a Canadian medical school with the desire to transfer to a United States medical school. This is possible but not probable. The competition for the few open spots in the United States is fierce just as it is in Canada. Most U.S. schools will have, at most, one or two open spots in the second, third, or fourth years, and applicants for these spots often have to be residents of the state where the school is located or a U.S. citizen. If a spot becomes open, the school wants to fill it, but they will do so with the most qualified candidate they can find. Transfer students will also usually have to take a series of competency tests on the basic sciences to prove that they have the ability to continue their education at that school. These tests are often held over the summer resulting in a loss of the vacation time that others will enjoy. It is also not uncommon for transfer students to be required to repeat the entire second year of the basic sciences at the school that has allowed the transfer. Step 1 USMLE® scores and AMRCB® certification will also be necessary for a transfer and the results of these tests should be exemplary. Some United States institutions may require that coursework taken at international institutions be evaluated for equivalence at United States institutions.

Many Canadian medical students and international medical graduates choose to take the United States Medical Licensing Examination (USMLE®) as well for various reasons. The following USMLE® information is provided for additional information for interested students.

UNITED STATES MEDICAL LICENSING EXAMINATION (USMLE®)

The USMLE® examination is a three step examination that is required for medical licensure in the United States. None of the USMLE® steps are required for medical licensure in Canada or by any medical schools located in Canada. All U.S Students are required to take USMLE® Step 1, USMLE® Step 2 - Clinical Knowledge, USMLE® Step 2 - Clinical Skills, and USMLE® Step 3. Canadian students who only desire to train and practice in Canada do not have any reason to take the USMLE®.

Canadian medical students take USMLE® for many different reasons. Common reasons include the desire to pursue a residency or fellowship in the United States, the desire to transfer into a U.S. medical school, or the desire to ultimately practice medicine in the U.S. For most U.S. residency programs, USMLE® Step 1 scores are very important in the residency application process. Many programs have a minimum USMLE® Step 1 score that is required before they are considered for a potential residency position. Not all U.S. fellowship programs require USMLE® scores, but some do, and the USMLE® is required if a physician desires to "moonlight" while in training. Nearly all states in the United States require the USMLE® to ultimately practice medicine, although California, Vermont, and New York will accept the Canadian licensing examination.

Many similarities are present between the USMLE® and the MCCEE. Both are multiple-choice examinations that have a patient problem presented in the question followed by multiple question choices related to the problem. While both tests address the basic sciences, the MCCEE does not explicitly test only the basic sciences assuming that this information must be known in order to answer the questions posed on the MCCEE. USMLE® Step 2 CK and the MCCEE both test the knowledge that is necessary for a physician to enter into supervised training, but there is variation in the questions based on physician tasks and the disease categories. The USMLE® Step 3 tests clinical knowledge for physicians entering medical practice which is different than material tested on the MCCEE. In addition, the scoring and procedures for reporting scores are different for both examinations.

In 1999, USMLE® Step 1 and USMLE® Step 2 were converted from a paper format to a computer-based format thus paper administrations of USMLE® Step 1 and USMLE® Step 2 are no longer available. The computer-based administrations are offered continuously at over 500 test centers worldwide.

USMLE® Step 1

USMLE® Step 1 is concerned with the basic medical sciences and assesses if a student can apply the understanding and knowledge of key concepts of the basic biomedical science. The mechanisms and principles of health, disease, and modes of therapy are assessed. Step 1 is the test used to demonstrate mastery of the basic sciences and that students have a basic foundation of this knowledge. Step 1 is usually taken at the end of the second year between the basic and clinical science years. The test is given over one day and consists of 322 multiple-choice questions and is divided into 7 blocks of 46 questions. It is a requirement by most schools that Step 1 is passed prior to beginning study of the clinical sciences. The current minimum passing score has been raised to 192, and has been raised several times over the last 2 decades.

USMLE® Step 2 Clinical Knowledge (CK)

USMLE® Step 2 Clinical Knowledge (CK) concentrates on the clinical sciences. This step assesses if a student can apply the medical knowledge and understanding of the clinical sciences, which is considered essential for providing patient care. Emphasis is placed on disease prevention, health promotion, and skills focused on caring for patients. The test is given over one day and can consist of varying numbers of questions and blocks, although the maximum amount of potential questions during the exam is 355 questions. The minimum passing score is 203 for Step 2 CK. Step 2 CK is usually taken at the end of the third or fourth year and is required by some schools prior to entering residency. Step 2 CK can, however, be taken at any time after passing USMLE® Step 1 providing eligibility requirements are met. Many students choose to take the USMLE® Step 2 CK at the beginning of the third year if they believe they can achieve a high score which would make them more competitive for residency. For those who do this, and score below average, this approach can backfire.

USMLE® Step 2 Clinical Skills (CS)

USMLE® Step 2 Clinical Skills (CS) is utilized to demonstrate the ability to provide patient care under supervision utilizing medical knowledge and the clinical sciences. Basic patient-focused care is stressed with the goal of being able to provide effective and safe care. Standardized patients are used as test subjects so that physical examinations and information gathering can be assessed. This test is currently graded on a pass/fail basis.

USMLE® Step 3

USMLE® Step 3 concentrates on general medical practice and the clinical sciences with the goal of demonstrating that a student can safely provide unsupervised medical care. The ambulatory care setting is stressed during this step with the overarching goal to reflect general clinical situations, although inpatient vignettes are used as well. The focus is on managing therapies and on the evaluation of patient problems. Multiple-choice questions and case simulations are utilized based on patient vignettes. This step is usually taken during the first year of residency but can be taken at any time during residency depending on the rules based on the state where the student has their training license. Individual states within the U.S. may have varying rules on when Step 3 can be taken depending on the citizenship and country where the medical education was obtained as well. Passing of Step 1, Step 2 CK, and Step 2 CS are prerequisites in order to take this test. Step 3 is generally considered the least difficult of the three steps and is taken over two days. Day one consists of 336 multiple-choice questions divided into seven blocks and day two consists of 144 multiple-choice questions divided over four blocks. Included in the second day is testing based upon case simulations which utilize a Primum® Tutorial which involves a 15-minute instructional period followed by testing based directly on twelve patient case presentations. The minimum passing score for Step 3 is 190.

The following tables display information on USMLE® performance for U.S and Canadian, and non-U.S. and Canadian test takers. Information for osteopathic trainees are included only if they have taken the USMLE®. Osteopathic physicians typically take the COMLEX® Steps 1, 2, and 3 and are not required to take the USMLE®. Many osteopathic students chose to take the USMLE®, however, in order to be more competitive for allopathic residencies and so that they can be compared directly with allopathic students who take only the USMLE® test series. It is noted that, in general, U.S. and Canadian medical school students score higher on USMLE® Step 1 on the initial attempt and when repeating the test than do non-U.S and Canadian students. This general trend holds true for USMLE® Step 2 CK, USMLE® Step 2 CS, and USMLE® Step 3. All subcomponent scores of the USMLE® Step 2 CS also note higher passing rates for U.S. and Canadian medical school students.

TABLE 7.3: Non-U.S. and Canadian School USMLE® Step 1 Performance

Non - U.S. and Canadian Schools	2012		2013	
	Number Tested	Percent Passing	Number Tested	Percent Passing
1st Attempt	14,201	76%	14,649	79%
Repeaters	4,261	40%	3,772	44%
Total	18,462	68%	18,421	72%

Source: Federation of State Medical Boards (FSMB) and National Board of Medical Examiners (NBME)

Table 7.4: U.S. and Canadian School USMLE® Step 1 Performance

U.S. and Canadian Schools	2012		2013	
	Number Tested	Percent Passing	Number Tested	Percent Passing
MD Degree	19,856	94%	20,023	95%
1st Attempt	18,723	96%	19,108	97%
Repeaters	1,133	68%	915	72%
DO Degree	2,564	91%	2,726	94%
1st Attempt	2,496	92%	2,680	94%
Repeaters	68	68%	46	74%
Total	22,420	94%	22,749	95%

Source: Federation of State Medical Boards (FSMB) and National Board of Medical Examiners (NBME)

TABLE 7.5: U.S. and Canadian School USMLE® Step 2 CK Performance

U.S. and Canadian Schools	2011-2012		2012-2013	
	Number Tested	Percent Passing	Number Tested	Percent Passing
MD Degree	18,929	97%	19,155	97%
1st Attempt	18,454	98%	18,658	98%
Repeaters	475	72%	497	74%
DO Degree	1,456	96%	1,634	96%
1st Attempt	1,439	97%	1,615	96%
Repeaters	17	53%	19	84%
Total	20,385	97%	20,789	97%

Source: Federation of State Medical Boards (FSMB) and National Board of Medical Examiners (NBME)

TABLE 7.6: Non-U.S. and Canadian School USMLE® Step 2 CK Performance

Non - U.S. and Canadian Schools	2011-2012		2012-2013	
	Number Tested	Percent Passing	Number Tested	Percent Passing
1st Attempt	11,908	85%	12,203	84%
Repeaters	2,191	54%	1,948	50%
Total	14,099	80%	14,151	80%

Source: Federation of State Medical Boards (FSMB) and National Board of Medical Examiners (NBME)

TABLE 7.7: Non-U.S. and Canadian School USMLE® Step 2 CS Performance

Non - U.S. and Canadian Schools	2011-2012		2012-2013	
	Number Tested	**Percent Passing**	**Number Tested**	**Percent Passing**
1st Attempt	11,515	80%	12,083	76%
Repeaters	2,265	65%	2,393	59%
Total	13,780	77%	14,476	73%

Source: Federation of State Medical Boards (FSMB) and National Board of Medical Examiners (NBME)

TABLE 7.8: U.S. and Canadian School USMLE® Step 2 CS Performance

U.S. and Canadian Schools	2011-2012		2012-2013	
	Number Tested	**Percent Passing**	**Number Tested**	**Percent Passing**
MD Degree	17,118	97%	20,201	97%
1st Attempt	16,662	97%	19,757	98%
Repeaters	456	92%	444	80%
DO Degree	46	87%	66	89%
1st Attempt	45	87%	63	89%
Repeaters	1	NA	3	NA
Total	17,164	97%	20,267	97%

Source: Federation of State Medical Boards (FSMB) and National Board of Medical Examiners (NBME)

TABLE 7.9: USMLE® Step 2 CS Subcomponent Passing Rates

Subcomponents:

Integrated Clinical Encounter (ICE), Communication and Interpersonal Skills (CIS), Spoken English Proficiency (SEP)

	2011-2012			2012-2013		
	ICE	CIS	SEP	ICE	CIS	SEP
All US/Canadian Schools	98%	99%	>99%	98%	99%	>99%
All Non-US/Canadian Schools	86%	89%	97%	81%	92%	97%

Source: Federation of State Medical Boards (FSMB) and National Board of Medical Examiners (NBME)

TABLE 7.10: U.S. and Canadian School USMLE® Step 3 Performance

U.S. and Canadian Schools	2012		2013	
	Number Tested	Percent Passing	Number Tested	Percent Passing
MD Degree	19,056	95%	19,886	96%
1st Attempt	18,172	96%	19,086	97%
Repeaters	884	69%	800	78%
DO Degree	16	100%	25	92%
1st Attempt	16	100%	23	96%
Repeaters	0	N/A	2	NA
Total	19,072	95%	19,911	96%

Source: Federation of State Medical Boards (FSMB) and National Board of Medical Examiners (NBME)

TABLE 7.11: Non-U.S. and Canadian School USMLE® Step 3 Performance

Non - U.S. and Canadian Schools	2012		2013	
	Number Tested	Percent Passing	Number Tested	Percent Passing
1st Attempt	8,500	83%	8,781	87%
Repeaters	2,006	56%	1,978	64%
Total	10,506	78%	10,759	83%

Source: Federation of State Medical Boards (FSMB) and National Board of Medical Examiners (NBME)

TABLE 7.12: International Medical Student 2012 USMLE® Step 1 Performance

	Step 1	Step 2 CK	Step 2 CS
U.S. Citizen First Attempt	3983	3151	3343
U.S. Citizen Repeaters	1676	854	488
International Citizen First Attempt	10,184	8761	8175
International Citizen Repeaters	2587	1337	1781

Source: Federation of State Medical Boards (FSMB) and National Board of Medical Examiners (NBME)

TABLE 7.13: Overall 2011-2012 USMLE® Step 1 and Step 2 Performance

	U.S. and Canadian Students	International Medical Students
Step 1 First Attempt	96%	76%
Step 1 Repeaters	68%	40%
Step 2 CK First Attempt	98%	85%
Step 2 CK Repeaters	71%	54%
Step 2 CS First Attempt	97%	80%
Step 2 CS Repeaters	92%	65%

Source: Federation of State Medical Boards (FSMB) and National Board of Medical Examiners (NBME)

Chapter 8

Residency

Obtaining a residency is the most important step in the journey of becoming a practicing physician. The medical degree can be earned anywhere, but without a residency, the goal of practicing medicine in Canada will not be possible. The quest for a Canadian residency position will be more difficult for physicians trained outside of Canada, but it is still possible. One of the primary reasons for the large number of internationally trained physicians who practice in Canada is the unmet need across the country. Large inflows of physicians currently migrate into Canada from India, Pakistan, Eastern Europe, and the Philippines.

Needless to say, competition is fierce, and any applicant desiring a residency position must have outstanding qualifications. Success is ultimately decided on personal abilities, references from the hospitals where the clinical clerkship rotations were completed, grades in medical school, standardized test scores, AMRCB® certification, and how well the student interviews for the residency on the phone and/or in person.

In Canada, medical graduates may enter into residency education after graduation of a three or four year medical school program. Medical residencies are also referred to as postgraduate medical education as well. Residency training is the final stage in the educational process required to become a fully licensed, practicing physician.

Different medical specialties have varying lengths of time required to complete training. Family medicine is a 2-year training program. Students may choose an optional third year to complete advanced training in emergency medicine, geriatric medicine, or other skills. Other medical and surgical specialties span three to five years with additional training required to complete surgical subspecialties.

Physicians who complete residency then challenge varying certification examinations to achieve Board Certification in specific medical specialties. Family physicians certify with the College of Family Physicians. Physicians who complete training in Medicine and Surgery certify with the Royal College of Physicians and Surgeons of Canada.

The residency training process is Canada is very similar to residency training in the United States. Although there is some variation in nomenclature, students enter into the first year internship in both countries and perform the same duties despite more formality with this in Canada. Physicians often choose subspecialty training much earlier in Canada than they do in the United States. Some specialties such as Cardiac Surgery which are entered into only after several years of training in the United States are direct entry programs in Canada. Although collective agreements are in place regarding work hours for residents in Canada, there are no direct national guidelines currently in place like there are in the United States.

Licensed and practicing physicians in Canada must maintain competency and training throughout their career. This is done through course work, additional training, research, writing, teaching, small-group learning, conference attendance, and study. This is traditionally called Continuing Medical Education (CME). Specific disciplines have "Maintenance of Certification" or "Maintenance of Proficiency" that provides specific guidelines for obtaining CME training.

Table: 8.1 - Length of Medical Residency Length in Canada

Medical Residency Length in Canada	
Family Medicine	2 years
Emergency Medicine Maternal Care Geriatric Medicine Palliative Care Sports Medicine	3 years
Internal Medicine Pediatrics	4 years
Psychiatry	5 years
Cardiac Surgery Neurosurgery General Surgery	6 years

CANADIAN RESIDENT MATCHING SERVICE

Medical graduates in Canada obtain a medical residency position through the Canadian Resident Matching Service (CaRMS). On average, 10-11 medical residency positions are available in Canada for every ten medical students in Canada. This ratio results in relatively few positions available to medical graduates from outside the Canadian system. Several medical schools do, though, dedicate a number of residency positions for IMG's. IMG's may apply for residency positions that are unfilled midway during the CaRMS match timeline as well.

The CaRMS is licensed from the National Matching Service Inc. (NMS) based in Canada. NMS has been providing matching services in North America over the last 50 years. The algorithm used in the match is known as the Roth-Peranson algorithm and was designed by the NMS president Elliott Peranson and Alvin Roth who both received the Nobel Prize in economics in 2012 based in part on the algorithm. CaRMS publishes detailed information on the Canadian match statistics each year.

Prospective residency applicants enter into the CaRMS process in the fall and eventually provide a rank order list of desired programs after interviewing during the interview season. Medical residency programs also provide a rank order of applicants during the same time period. The rank order lists of both are then combined through the algorithm which results in the final rank orders lists for the country. Both lists are confidential. Applicants are placed into their most preferred program with the list of the applicants as the primary source driving the outcome. The algorithm attempts to match all applicants until such time as no more possibilities exist at which time the applicant would remain unmatched. Students are notified in March of the outcome and match.

CaRMS recommends the following guidelines for preparation of an applicant rank order list:

- Applicants should rank the programs that represent their true preferences in sequence.

- Applicants should consider the competitiveness of the specialty, the competitiveness of the programs, and the overall qualifications that an applicant has when determining the number of programs to rank

- All acceptable programs for the applicant should be ranked, and all unacceptable programs should not be ranked.

INTERNATIONAL MEDICAL GRADUATES (IMG'S) AND CANADIANS STUDYING ABROAD (CSA'S) IN CANADA

The number of IMG's matched into Canadian medical residencies has grown over the last 15 years increasing by over 500%. Over 1000 residency positions have been added over the last decade in Canada primarily for Canadian medical graduates, with 388 additional residency positions dedicated to IMG's. Despite this increase, due to the overall number of IMG's applying for these spots, the overall percentage of IMG's matching into residency positions in Canada has decreased. In 2000, only 77 IMG's were in residency training in Canada. By 2012, the Canadian Post-MD Education Registry (CAPER) reported 465 IMG's in Canadian post-graduate training. In 2012, 15% of first year residents were IMGs, while only 5% of first year residents were IMG's in 2000. During 2012, over 2,200 IMG's were in postgraduate training programs throughout Canada.

CaRMS reports data that notes that the numbers of IMG's applying for Canadian residencies has increased. Just over 1,500 IMG's applied to residency programs in 2008. Of these, 88% were IMG's and 12% were Canadians Studying Abroad (CSA's). Of these, 58% of the CSA's matched while only 25% of the IMG's matched to residency positions. By 2011, 25% of those applying through the CaRMS were CSA's with the remaining 75% consisting of IMG's. For 2011, 14% of CSA's matched, while only 14% of IMG's matched into a residency position. On average, over 400 IMG's enter into residency programs in Canada each year.

Current initiatives are underway in the country to aid in improving the process of IMG's matching into residency positions. The National Assessment Collaboration (NAC) is in place to provide a national approach to the assessment of the clinical skills and medical knowledge of IMG's. The NAC examination has been recommended to be the first step for IMG's who desire to enter the Canadian system. The NAC examination is considered to be fair in evaluating both CSA's and IMG's. Multiple groups and associations are in place which lobbies on behalf of CSA's, IMG's or both groups equally. Individual Canadian provinces do still have additional steps for IMG's such as Alberta who requires that an IMG has their credentials verified by an International Qualification Assessment Services. Agreements for national standards and several mutual recognition agreements are either in existence or being formed across different provinces. The Royal College of Physicians and Surgeons of Canada have a Practice Ready Assessment Route in place for IMG's who desire to live and work in Canada. The College of Family Physicians of Canada has a process in place to confer certification for physicians trained outside of Canada.

Many Canadian physicians work in countries other than Canada as well. Over 8,500 are currently practicing in the United States. Many others are practicing medicine in the United Kingdom, throughout Europe, Australia, Asia, as well as other locations. Overall, the retention of physicians in Canada has been difficult over the last two decades hovering between 86-93%. The overall number appears to have stabilized over the last several years.

CANADIANS STUDYING MEDICINE ABROAD

Despite an increase in medical school enrollment across Canada over the last 13 years, Canada still has the lowest ratio of doctors to patients of any first-world nation. Many Canadians have chosen to study and practice in countries other than their home country for various reasons. Regardless of the reason, this is an option to receive medical training for those struggling to gain acceptance to Canadian medical schools. It is estimated that if all graduates from international medical schools each year who were Canadian citizens were to return to Canada to practice, that this would equal over 750 new physicians each year. As of 2010, over 80 medical schools located in 30 countries reported having Canadian students enrolled in their medical education programs. Many programs are taught in English such as those in the Caribbean region, although many are taught in the language of the country where the education is received. Nearly half of all Canadians studying abroad do so in the Caribbean.

The cost of an international education can be high, and Canadians who study abroad have nearly $100,000 CAD in debt more than students studying in Canada. International graduates can choose to study in any field with the largest percentage matching into Family Medicine (21%). It is reported that nearly 90% want to return to Canada to practice, but the majority are often not able to complete this for several reasons. Limited residency positions; real and perceived barriers; the requirement of "return for service"; the choice of disciplines not being available; and the lack of believing that the student had a reasonable chance to practice back in Canada are all commonly cited.

The demographics of Canadians studying abroad note that slightly more than half were male; they were older than the average student in Canada; over 83% were single, divorced, or separated; students were more often children of physicians; and the majority come from Ontario and British Columbia. Approximately 6% entered directly from high school and 27% never applied to a Canadian medical school. More of these students have advanced degrees in comparison with Canadian students. Students studying abroad applied an average of 2.6 times to Canadian medical schools as opposed to 1.7 times by successful Canadian students. A consistent problem for international students is in arranging for Canadian rotations in the clerkship years. Canadian students in Australia and Ireland were the most successful in securing clerkship rotations in Canada.

Of the Canadians studying abroad, over 90% had obtained at least part of their post-secondary education in Canada prior to going to medical school abroad. The motivation reported for studying abroad to the CaRMS study in 2010 noted the inability to place into a medical school in Canada. The fact that students could enter directly after secondary school education and the fact that tuition costs were lower abroad were important as well. In addition, students also reported wanting to live in another country and that their family was in/from the country where they were going to study. Students selected medical school's abroad based on the school's reputation; the likelihood of obtaining North American clerkships; the language of instruction; cost; proximity to Canada; and the attractiveness of the country. Over 70% of students funded their education with family savings or bank loans.

Table 8.2: Canadian Students Studying Abroad

Region of Medical School	Number Enrolled Canadians
Australia	550
Caribbean	2000
Ireland	650
Middle East	70
Poland	300
Total*	3570

Source: Canadian students Studying Medicine Abroad. CaRMS 2010
* Other includes China, Central America, and South America

International Medical Schools

Many students from international countries attend medical schools in the Caribbean, Central America, and South America for various reasons. The advantage of attending a Caribbean, Central American, or South American medical school instead of other international medical schools is that many of these schools are able to place their students in affiliated hospitals in the United States and Canada during clinical rotations in the third and fourth year. Residency programs often feel more comfortable with students that have been trained in Canadian and United States hospitals and are thus familiar with the medical technology and procedures in North America. Students who have performed clinical rotations in North America will benefit from making contacts and friendships with supervisors and other physicians. These relationships will allow the student to obtain letters of reference that can aid a student in obtaining a residency position.

Caribbean, Central American, and South American medical schools also place many students in residencies throughout other areas across the globe according to differing criteria. Some students are placed by choice and availability, but the students placed in Canada and the United States are done so usually as a result of competition and grades. The overarching goal of most schools is to place students in North America for clinical rotations. Certain hospitals, specialties, and geographic areas will be highly competitive while others will offer a much greater chance of placement.

For an internationally trained physician, performance throughout the undergraduate and graduate education is very important when it comes to obtaining a residency. Standardized test scores and AMRCB® certification are the most important as this shows competency and abilities in comparison to the students trained in Canada and the United States. An aspiring physician trained in the Caribbean, Central America, and South America with above average standardized test scores and AMRCB® certification will be well on their way toward obtaining a North American residency.

Canadian Medical Schools

Seventeen medical schools operate in Canada. Thirteen schools provide instruction in English, three provide instruction in French (Laval, Montreal, and Sherbrooke) and one school provides bilingual instruction (Ottawa). Two programs are three years in length (McMaster and Calgary) with the remaining schools providing instruction over four year.

Alberta

- University of Alberta, Faculty of Medicine and Dentistry
- University of Calgary, Cumming School of Medicine

British Columbia

- University of British Columbia, Faculty of Medicine

Manitoba

- University of Manitoba, Faculty of Medicine

Newfoundland

- Memorial University of Newfoundland, Faculty of Medicine

Nova Scotia

- Dalhousie University, Faculty of Medicine

Ontario

- McMaster University, Michael G. DeGroote School of Medicine
- Northern Ontario School of Medicine
- University of Ottawa, Faculty of Medicine
- Queen's University, School of Medicine
- University of Toronto, Faculty of Medicine
- Western University, Schulich School of Medicine and Dentistry

Quebec

- Université Laval, Faculté de médecine
- McGill University, Faculty of Medicine
- Université de Montréal, Faculté de médecine
- Université de Sherbrooke, Faculté de médecine

Saskatchewan

- University of Saskatchewan, College of Medicine

Information in this publication has come directly from individual medical school websites, catalogues, and the Office of Research and Information Services (ORIS). A significant amount of information was obtained directly from the AFMC publication titled; *Admission Requirements of Canadian Faculties of Medicine - Admission in 2015*. Information is subject to change each year.

Alberta

University of Alberta, Faculty of Medicine and Dentistry

University of Calgary, Cumming School of Medicine

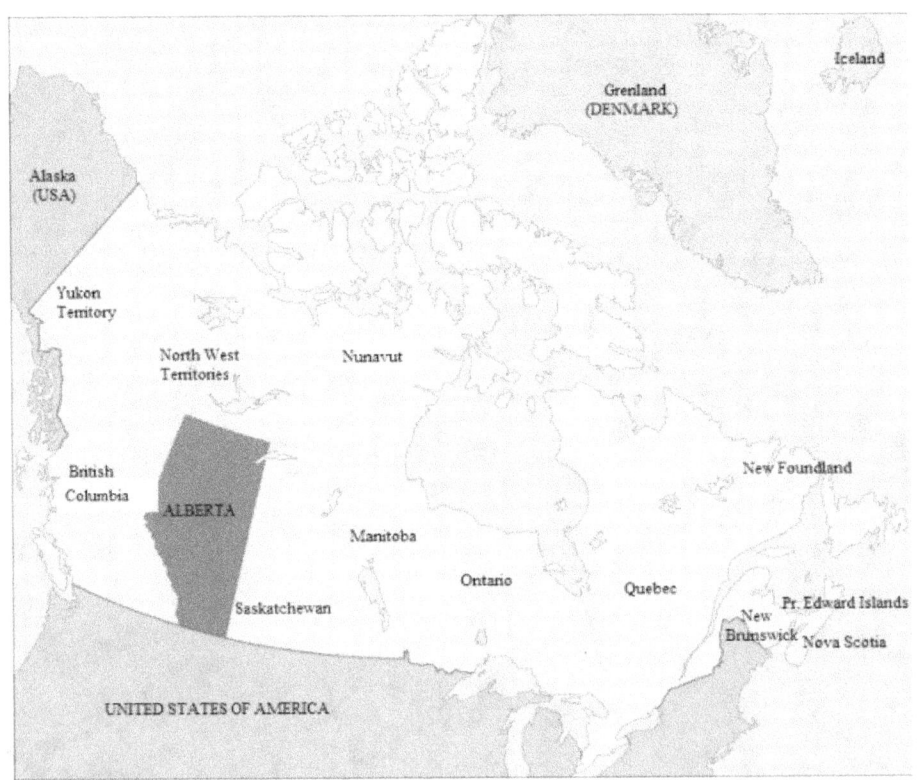

University of Alberta, Faculty of Medicine and Dentistry

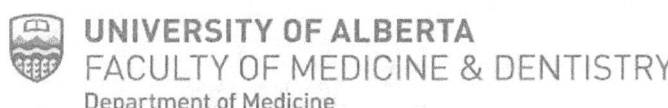

UNIVERSITY OF ALBERTA
FACULTY OF MEDICINE & DENTISTRY
Department of Medicine

QUICK FACTS

POSITIONS:
167: Total
25: Out-of-province
10: Rural
5: Aboriginal

Class: 85% Alberta residents
Average age of 1st year: 23
Male/Female %: 56/44

UNIVERSITY:
Type: Public

APPLICATIONS:
Accept Non-Canadians: No
Transfers: No
Deferred Admissions: No

Primary Application:
Electronic - School Specific

Secondary Application: Yes

Early Decision: Yes

CURRICULUM:
Length: 4-years
Language: English

Douglas Miller - Dean, Faculty of Medicine & Dentistry, University of Alberta

CAMPUS:
Admissions Office
Undergraduate Medical Education
Faculty of Medicine & Dentistry
University of Alberta
1-002 Katz Group Centre for Pharmacy
and Health Research
Edmonton AB T6G 2E1

CONTACT INFORMATION:
Telephone: 780-492-6350 or 492-9531
Fax: 780-492-9531

E-Mail: ume.general@ualberta.ca
Website: http://www.med.ualberta.ca/

GENERAL INFORMATION:

The University of Alberta was founded in 1913 and now consists of 20 departments with multiple research groups and institutions. The school emphasizes research and clinical care and has several joint degrees. The mission is dedicated to the improvement of health through excellence and leadership in the educational programs, in fundamental and applied research, and in the prevention and treatment of illness. The University of Alberta seeks to prepare physicians to provide the highest quality of health care to the people of Alberta and beyond, and to advance knowledge and its application through research. The University is committed to a tradition of excellence in all programs according to national and international standards.

The goals of the school are to develop and deliver the highest quality of educational programs in medicine and related health sciences. The University seeks to provide outstanding clinical leadership and professional consultation in the provision of medical services and the development of healthcare programs. The objective of the MD program is to develop collaborative, compassionate, knowledgeable, reflective, and professional physicians who are committed to quality health care and life-long learning. The University is dedicated to provide a learner-centric model of education.

Campus housing is available.

PREREQUISITES:

Two full years of academic study is required prior to applying.

Required Courses (laboratory work with science coursework is expected):

AP/IB: May claim some credit for Biology, English, General Chemistry, Physics, and Statistics

General Chemistry – 1 year	Organic Chemistry – 1 year	Biology – 1 year
Physics – 1 year	English – 1 year	Statistics - ½ year
Biochemistry – ½ year		

Testing of Language Proficiency: Yes
MCAT® Required: Yes
AMRCB® transcripts: Send via direct mail

<u>MCAT®</u>

MCAT Required: Yes

Average MCAT: 33

Average MCAT Bio: 10.8
Average MCAT Phys: 11.3
Average MCAT Verbal: 11.37
Average MCAT Essay: Q

MCAT minimum:
Alberta Residents: 7 any category

Non-Alberta Residents: 11-Verbal   7- All others

<u>GPA:</u>

3.91: GPA (overall)
3.3: GPA (minimum)

3.3: Alberta Resident minimum GPA

3.5: Non-Alberta Resident minimum GPA

<u>Preparatory Programs:</u>

Summer: No

Post-baccalaureate: no

<u>Combined Programs:</u>

MD/MBA, MD/PhD, MD (with Special Training in Research)

CURRICULUM:

Basic Sciences:

Multiple learning processes are utilized to include lectures, problem-based learning, computer-based study, independent study, and laboratory work. The school desires to educate students in an interdisciplinary environment of learning, research, public services, and practice. The curriculum is given over 35 weeks and takes place primarily at the medical sciences building.

Basic Sciences

Year 1	Year 2
Introduction to Medicine and Dentistry	Gastroenterology and Nutrition
Infection, Immunity and Inflammation	Reproductive Medicine and Urology
Endocrinology and Metabolism	Musculoskeletal System
Cardiovascular, Pulmonary and Renal Systems	Neurosciences
Physicianship	Oncology
Interprofessional Health Team Development	Patient-Centered Care, Part II
Electives – 12 hours	

Clinical Sciences:

The Clinical Sciences are focused primarily on developing clinical skills which are taught primarily during the clerkships and supported by some classroom instruction. In addition to the Clerkships, students participate in an Integrated Community Clerkship of 36 weeks during the third year. A review course, skills lab, and ACLS course are also part of the clinical years.

Training takes place primarily at University of Alberta hospitals, Cross Cancer Institute, Edmonton General Hospital, Glenrose Hospital, Grey Nuns Hospital, Misericordia Hospital, and the Royal Alexandra Hospital. A limited number of electives can be arranged at non-affiliated hospitals.

Clinical Skills

Required Clerkships	Electives and Selectives
Medicine – 8 weeks	Electives – 13 weeks
Family Medicine – 8 weeks	
Pediatrics – 8 weeks	Surgery – 6 weeks
Surgery – 6 weeks	
Psychiatry – 6 weeks	
OB/GYN – 6 weeks	
Emergency Medicine – 3 weeks	
Geriatrics – 3 weeks	

Thesis/Research Required: Optional
Community Service Requirements: Required - rural Family Medicine training.

TUITION: All currency listings are in Canadian Dollars (CAD)

Canadian Residents: $12,756
Compulsory Fees: $1,260

Application Fee:
$75 for Alberta undergraduates
$125 for all others.

Applicants complete the undergraduate application first, followed by a secondary medicine application.
Acceptance Deposit: $1,000 (non-refundable) – applied toward tuition

INTERVIEW:

Interviews: Multiple Mini Interviews (MMI) take place in March each year. A total of 473 applicants were interviewed in 2014. Of these, 408 were Alberta residents and 65 were non-Alberta residents.

Acceptance Notification: Mailed in May each year.

SELECTION FACTORS:

Academic Criteria:
Two years of full-time university/college is required. The minimum acceptable grade point average on a 4.0 scale is 3.3 for Alberta residents; 3.5 for non-Alberta residents with 4 or more years post-secondary study; and 3.7 for students with 2 or 3 years post-secondary study (not receiving a degree). The mean grade point average of successful applicants in 2013/14 was 3.91.

The MCAT® is required and the test must have been taken no later than September, 2014 and no earlier than October, 2009. The minimum acceptable MCAT® score for Alberta residents is 7 in any category. The minimum MCAT® score for non-Alberta residents is 11 in Verbal Reasoning and 7 in each of Physical Sciences and Biological Sciences.

The Admissions Committee seeks to build a diverse class. It is recommended that students highlight their positive life experiences. Many areas are considered including an applicant's leadership roles, awards, employment records, diversity of experience, and volunteer work. Additional credit for applicants is awarded for those with Master's and PhD degrees. The personal interviews are an important part of the selection process.

Table 1: University of Alberta Applicant Match Statistics^*

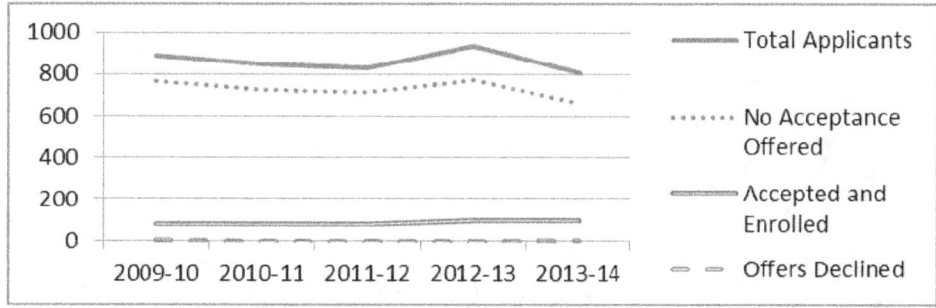

^ Success rate is defined as the percentage of applicants receiving at least one offer of admission regardless of acceptance
* Includes Canadian citizens/landed immigrants who were living outside Canada at time of application
Source: Admission Requirements of Canadian Faculties of Medicine

Table 2: University of Alberta Applicant Selection Success

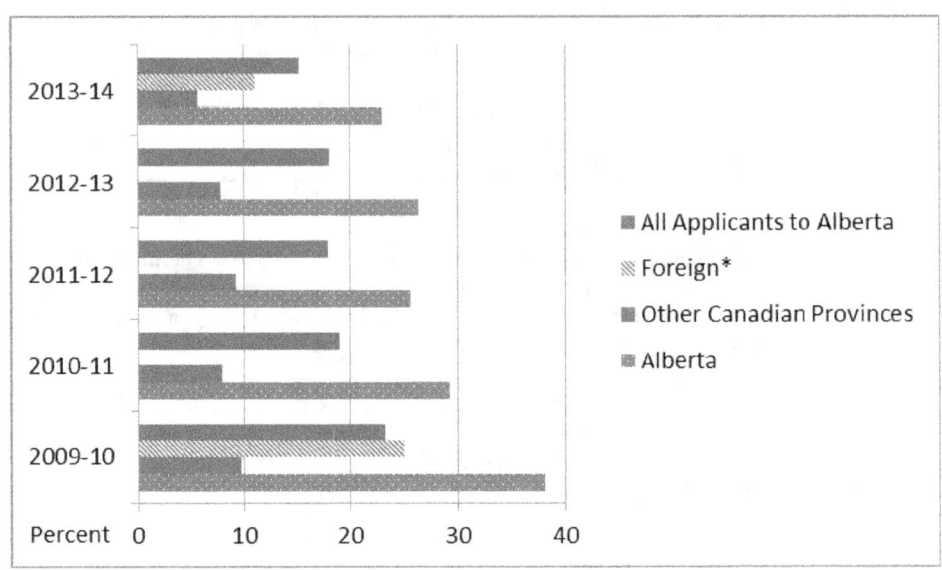

Source: Admission Requirements of Canadian Faculties of Medicine

University of Calgary, Cumming School of Medicine

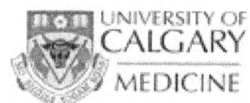

QUICK FACTS

POSITIONS:
170: Total
25: Out-of-province and Aboriginal

85%: Alberta Residents
Average age of 1st year: 25.2
Male/Female %: 47/53

UNIVERSITY:
Type: Public

APPLICATIONS:
Accept Non-Canadians: No
Transfers: No
Deferred Admissions: Yes

Primary Application: UCAN Electronic - School Specific

Secondary Application: No

Early Decision: No

CURRICULUM:
Length: 3-years
Language: English

Dr. Jon Meddings - Dean, Cumming School of Medicine

CAMPUS:
Office of Admissions
Faculty of Medicine
University of Calgary
3330 Hospital Drive NW
Calgary AB T2N 4N1

CONTACT INFORMATION:
Telephone: 403-220-4262
Fax: 403-210-8148

E-Mail: ucmedapp@ucalgary.ca
Website: www.ucalgary.ca/mdprogram

GENERAL INFORMATION:

The University of Calgary was founded in 1970 and has been at the current location since 1972. The mission of the school is to shape the future of society, be responsive to community and societal needs, to be rooted in basic research and discovery, and to be committed to excellence, innovation, and creativity.

The curriculum is a three-year curriculum that is rigorous by design spanning 11 months each year. Several combined degree program are available. The curriculum is called the Clinical Presentation Curriculum and focuses on system-based learning. The University is committed to rural social accountability and students participate in rural rotations.

Campus Housing; On Campus for married and single students is available

PREREQUISITES:

Two years of full-time university study is required prior to applying.

No specific requirements are in place, although several courses are recommended. Recommended courses include: Anthropology, Biochemistry, Biology, Calculus, Chemistry, English, Organic Chemistry, Physics, Physiology, Sociology, and Statistics.

Testing of Language Proficiency: No
MCAT® Required: Yes
AMRCB® transcript: Send via direct mail

CURRICULUM:

Basic Sciences:

Coursework is based on organ systems and utilizes small group discussions and lectures. The curriculum is the Clinical Presentation Curriculum which teaches the Basic and Clinical Sciences as they pertain to individual clinical cases. Students participate in independent research projects during the two years of the Basic Sciences. Instructions take place in the Calgary Health Sciences Center which is less than a mile (1.5 km) from the

University of Calgary's main campus. Courses are designed as multidisciplinary units allowing for application of concepts from a systems perspective.

MCAT®

MCAT Required: Yes

Average Total MCAT: 31.8

Average MCAT Bio: 10.9
Average MCAT Phys: 10.3
Average MCAT Verbal: 10.6
Average MCAT Essay: Q

Minimum MCAT scores: 8 in any category

GPA:

3.82: GPA (overall)

3.2: Alberta Resident minimum GPA

3.8: Non-Alberta Resident minimum GPA

Combined Programs:

MD/PhD, MD/MBA, MD/MSc, MD/MA

Basic Sciences

Year 1	Year 2
Intro to Medicine/Blood/Gastrointestinal	Renal/Endocrine/Obesity
Musculoskeletal and Skin	Neuroscience/Aging/Special Senses
Cardiology/Respirology	Children's and Women's Health
Population Health	Psychiatry
Family Medicine Clinical Experience	Applied Evidence Based Medicine
Medical Skills	Medical Skills
History of Medicine	Introduction to Clinical Practice

Clinical Sciences:

Clinical training takes place at the Alberta Children's Clinic, Foothills Hospital, the Peter Lougheed Center, Rockyview Hospital., and the University of Calgary Medical Clinic. Students participate in rural rotations at several sites including Medicine Hat, Lethbridge, Red Deer, Yellowknife, and other rural sites such as Brooks, High Level, and Pincher Creek. Students generally spend 5–10 weeks of their clinical rotations in rural locations. Community service is not required, but is strongly recommended.

Clinical Skills

Required Clerkships	Electives and Selectives
Internal Medicine – 12 weeks Surgery – 8 weeks Psychiatry – 6 weeks Pediatrics – 6 weeks OB/GYN – 6 weeks Family Medicine – 4 weeks Anesthesia – 2 weeks	Electives – 10 weeks

Thesis/Research Required: Optional
Community Service Requirements: Optional, but strongly recommended

TUITION: All currency listings are in Canadian Dollars (CAD)

Canadian Residents: $15,012   Foreign Students: $65,000
Compulsory Fees: $793

Application Fee:$150
Acceptance Deposit: $500 (non-refundable) – applied toward tuition

INTERVIEW:

Interviews: Take place in February each year. A total of 539 applicants were interviewed in 2014. Of these, 450 were residents of Alberta and 89 were residents in other areas of Canada. Applicants of Aboriginal descent are automatically interviewed if they meet the minimum grade point average.

Acceptance Notification: Mailed in May each year.

SELECTION FACTORS:

An internal admission score is develop for each applicant based on college coursework, MCAT® scores, and the interview. The MCAT® is required and must have been taken after 1991. The internal admission score cut-off is higher for those not from Alberta to be offered an interview, although the cut-off scores to be offered acceptance is historically the same for those from Alberta as those from other locations in Canada. The Admissions Committee seeks to identify applicants with the professional skills and maturity required to be a successful physician. Leadership and altruism are necessary traits for physicians and these traits are sought in applicants. Although no specific prerequisite coursework is in place for applicants, students should be accomplished academically and have demonstrated academic success in all coursework. Special attention is given to success in science coursework. Letters of recommendation are important in identifying motivated applicants. Additional consideration is given to aboriginal applicants.

Table 1: University of Calgary Applicant Match Statistics^*

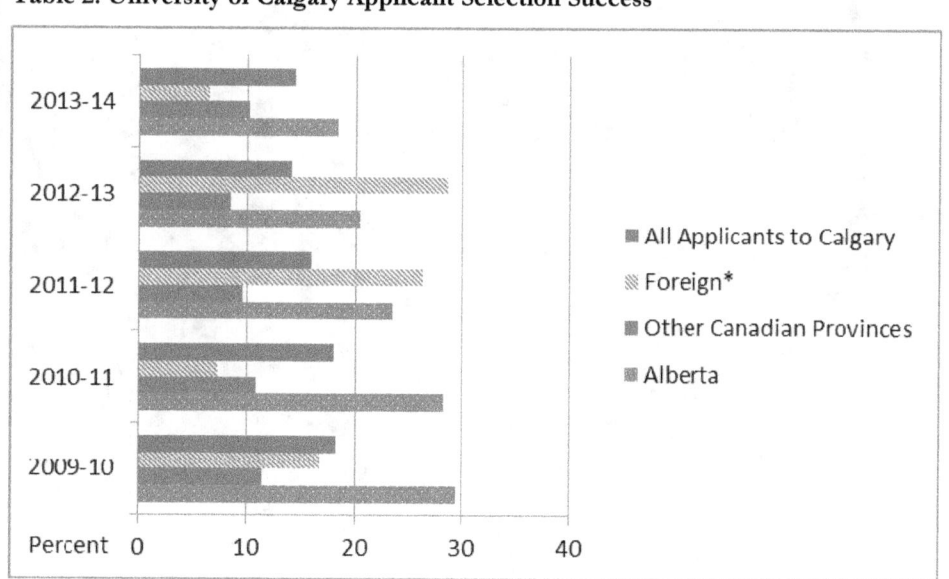

^ Success rate is defined as the percentage of applicants receiving at least one offer of admission regardless of acceptance
* Includes Canadian citizens/landed immigrants who were living outside Canada at time of application
Source: Admission Requirements of Canadian Faculties of Medicine

Table 2: University of Calgary Applicant Selection Success

Source: Admission Requirements of Canadian Faculties of Medicine

British Columbia

University of British Columbia, Faculty of Medicine

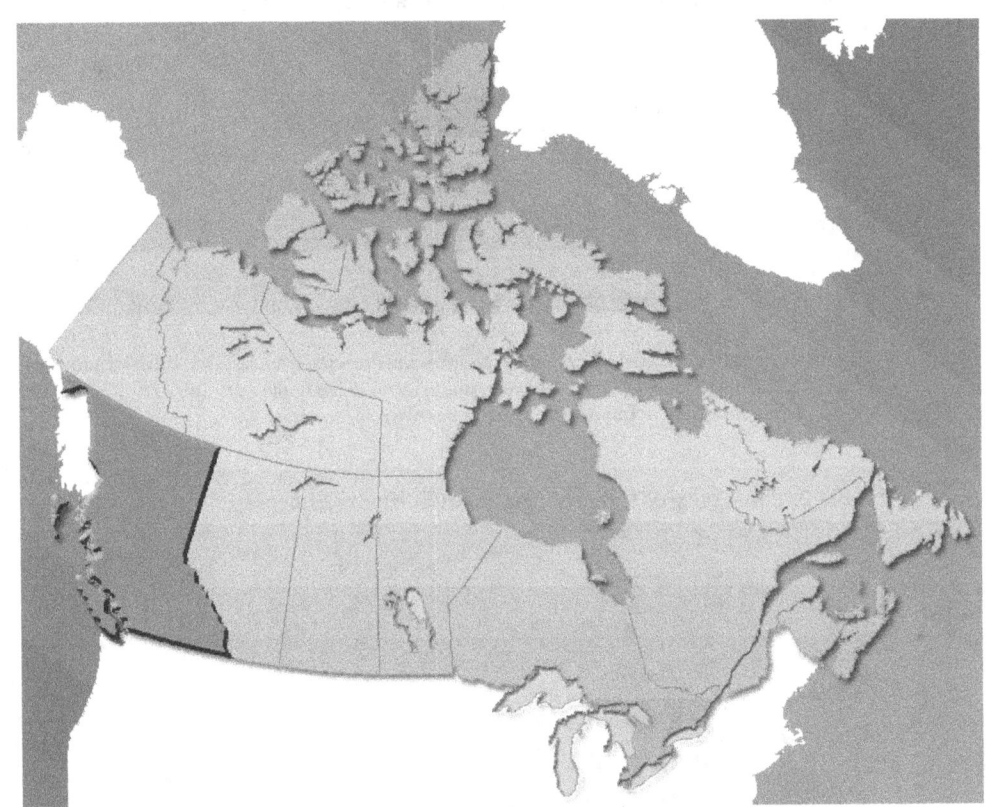

University of British Columbia, Faculty of Medicine

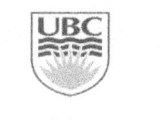

FACULTY OF MEDICINE

QUICK FACTS

POSITIONS:
288: Total
29: Out-of-Province
14: Aboriginal
5: MD/PhD

Average age of 1st year: 23

UNIVERSITY:
Type: Public

APPLICATIONS:
Accept Non-Canadians: No
Transfers: Yes
Deferred Admissions: Yes

Primary Application:
Electronic - School Specific

Secondary Application: Yes

Early Decision: No

CURRICULUM:
Length: 4-years
Language: English

Dr. Gavin Stuart- Dean, Faculty of Medicine

CAMPUS:
University of British Columbia
Faculty of Medicine, Dean's Office
MD Undergraduate Admissions
317-2194 Health Sciences Mall
Vancouver BC V6T 1Z3

CONTACT INFORMATION:
Telephone: 604-822-2421
Fax: 604-822-6061

E-Mail: admission.md@ubc.ca
Website: mdprogram.med.ubc.ca

GENERAL INFORMATION:

The University of British Columbia was founded in 1908 and prepares students for practice in the 21st Century. The University expanded in 2004 and is now operating four campuses and is one of the largest medical schools in North America. The main campus is the Frasier Medical Program in Vancouver which instructs 192 students. The Island medical Program in Victoria, the Northern Medical Program in Prince George, and the Southern Medical Program in Kelowna all host 32 students each. All positions at all locations are filled based on the same selection process. Students are assigned to the Northern Medical Campus based on a suitability tool used for the rural and remote areas. Applicants select a site preference during the interview process.

The goal of the school is to provide learning environments that are conducive to learning and effective knowledge acquisition. The mission of the school is to recruit, admit, educate, and support students who will graduate with defined and demonstrated personal qualities. The university focuses on the competencies, knowledge, and behaviors rooted in the vision, missions, and values of the institution.

The curriculum is designed to be comprehensive and integrated and utilizes small group problem-based learning. Students are expected to be strong collaborators and self-directed in their education. Graduate programs and combined degrees are available as is a post-baccalaureate preparatory program.

On Campus housing is available.

PREREQUISITES:

Three years of full-time study is required.

AP/IB: Can claim credit for Biology, English, and Chemistry with high exam grades

Required Courses (laboratory work with science coursework is expected):

General Chemistry – 1 year	Organic Chemistry – 1 year	Biology – 1 year
English – 1 year	Biochemistry – 1 year	

Several options are available as alternate methods to meet the one year Biochemistry requirement.

Although not required, courses in behavioral sciences, biometrics, statistics and physics are recommended.

Testing of Language Proficiency: No
MCAT® Required: Yes
AMRCB® transcript: Send via direct mail

MCAT®

MCAT Required: Yes

Average MCAT: 3.0

Average MCAT Bio: 10.4
Average MCAT Phys: 10.1
Average MCAT Verbal: 9.5
Average MCAT Essay: Q

MCAT Minimum: 7/7/7/M

GPA:

3.82 GPA(overall)
2.8: GPA (minimum)

Combined Programs:

MD/PhD

CURRICULUM:

Basic Sciences:

Learning takes place using a case-based curriculum. Small group forums, lectures, laboratories, and computer-based instruction are also utilized. The program is built on the principles of self-directed learning.

Basic Sciences

Year 1	Year 2
Foundations of Medicine -Host Defenses and Infection -Cardiovascular -Pulmonary -Fluids and Electrolytes, and Renal GU	Foundation of Medicine -Blood and Lymphatics -Gastrointestinal -Musculoskeletal and Locomotor -Endocrine and Metabolism -Integument -Brain and Behavior -Reproduction -Growth and Development
Principles of Human Biology	Doctor Patient and Society
Doctor Patient and Society	Family Practice Continuum
Family Practice Continuum	

Clinical Sciences:

Clinical training begins with courses in Health Care Epidemiology, Radiology, and Therapeutics. A four week orientation takes place prior to the start of the clerkships. Clinical training occurs at over 80 affiliated sites and includes British Columbia Cancer Center Agency; British Columbia Children's Hospital; British Columbia Woman's Hospital and Health Center; Canadian Arthritis and Rheumatism Society Center; G.F. Strong Rehabilitation Center; St. Paul's Hospital; University Hospital; and the Vancouver General Hospital.

Clinical Skills

Required Clerkships	Electives and Selectives
Medicine – 10 weeks Surgery – 8 weeks Psychiatry – 8 weeks Pediatrics – 8 weeks OB/GYN – 8 weeks Emergency Medicine – 4 weeks Rural Family Medicine – 4 weeks Anesthesia – 2 weeks Orthopedics – 2 weeks Dermatology – 1 week Ophthalmology – 1 week	Third Year Electives – 6 weeks Fourth Year Electives – 16 weeks

Thesis/Research Required: Optional
Community Service Requirements: Optional

TUITION: All currency listings are in Canadian Dollars (CAD)

Canadian Residents: $16,731
Compulsory Fees: $988

Application Fee: $111 for BC Residents with BC Transcripts
$143 for BC Residents with out-of-province transcripts
$164 for Non-BC Residents
Acceptance Deposit: $1,000 (non-refundable) – applied toward tuition

INTERVIEW:

Interviews: Take place in March each year and are conducted in a Mini-Interview format. A total of 654 applicants were interviewed in 2014. Of these, 573 were from British Columbia and 81 residents were from other location in Canada. Applicants are invited based on a file review of academic and non-academic qualifications.

Acceptance Notification: Mailed in May each year.

SELECTION FACTORS:

The Admissions Committee evaluates the overall personal characteristics of students and the overall academic qualifications. Academic qualifications are expected to be excellent. The motivations of students as well as an applicant's integrity are important factors. Students are expected to be mature, motivated, and to have a genuine concern for humanity. Creativity, social concern, intellectual curiosity, integrity, maturity, and attitude toward continuing learning are all valuable assets for applicants. The pool of applicants is highly competitive. The Admissions Committee seeks to recruit well-rounded, dedicated, intelligent students from diverse backgrounds. Letters of recommendation are considered strongly in the selection process. No specific preference is given to any specific undergraduate major.

The MCAT® is required and the test must have been taken within the last 5 years. All prerequisite science coursework must be completed at a minimum score of 70% and the vast majorities of students have scores much higher than this. A composite score is developed for an applicant that consists of the MCAT® score, GPA, the interview score, and non-academic activities. Several academic averages are determined including the overall academic average on all coursework attempted, the adjusted academic average which allows some grades to be dropped, and a prerequisite academic average. On average, one-third of applicants are invited for an interview.

Applications from well-qualified Aboriginal applicants are considered as are applications from those who desire to serve in a rural community. Applicants who self-identify as Aboriginal will be considered under the Aboriginal admission process as well as under the regular admission process

Table 1: University of British Columbia Applicant Match Statistics^*

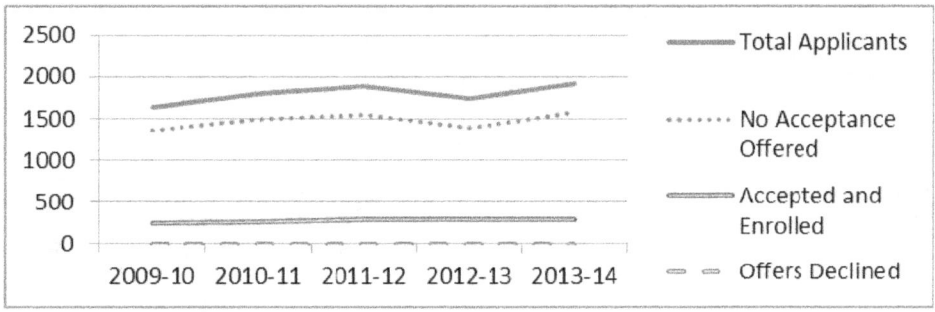

^ Success rate is defined as the percentage of applicants receiving at least one offer of admission regardless of acceptance
* Includes Canadian citizens/landed immigrants who were living outside Canada at time of application
Source: Admission Requirements of Canadian Faculties of Medicine

Table 2: University of British Columbia Applicant Selection Success

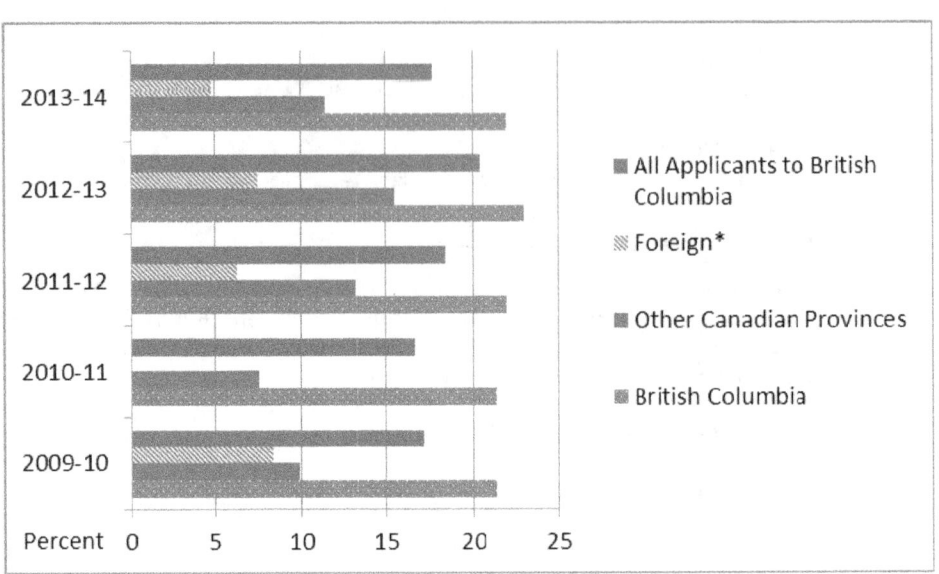

Source: Admission Requirements of Canadian Faculties of Medicine

Manitoba

University of Manitoba, Faculty of Medicine

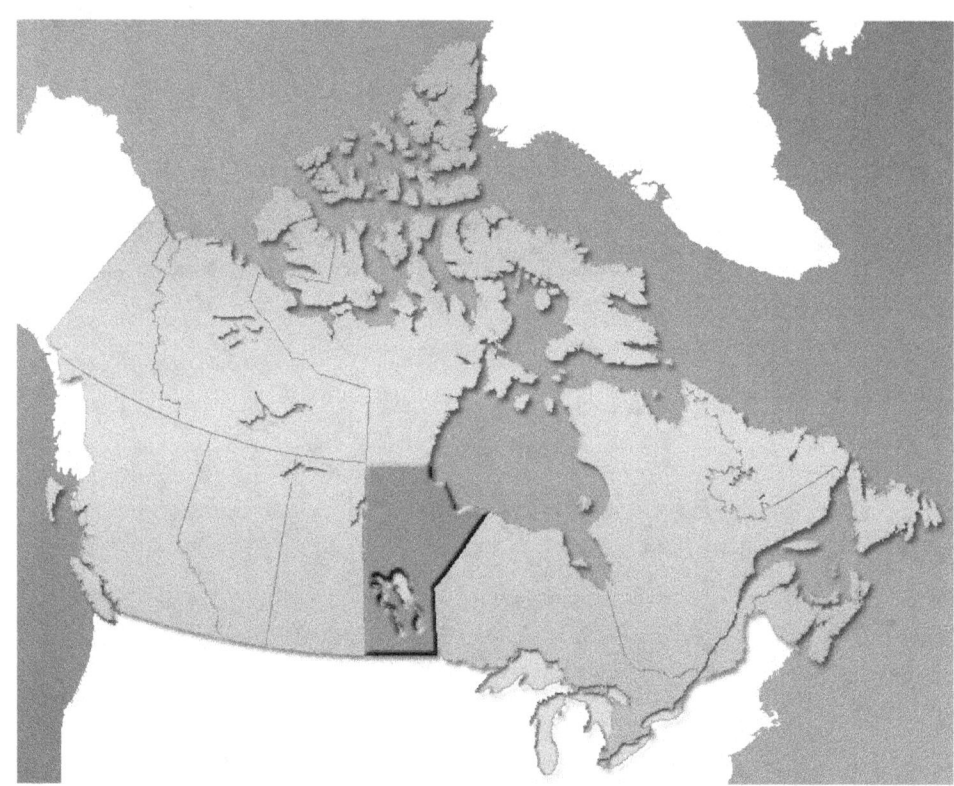

University of Manitoba, Faculty of Medicine

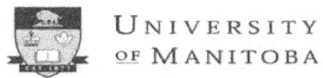

QUICK FACTS

POSITIONS:
110: Total
11: Out-of-province

Average age of 1st year: 24
Male/Female %: 51/49

UNIVERSITY:
Type: Public

APPLICATIONS:
Accept Non-Canadians: No
Transfers: Yes
Deferred Admissions: Yes

Primary Application:
Electronic - School Specific

Secondary Application: Yes

Early Decision: No

CURRICULUM:
Length: 4-years
Language: English

Dr. Brian Postl - Dean, Faculty of Medicine

CAMPUS:
Admissions
Faculty of Medicine
University of Manitoba
S204, 750 Bannatyne Ave
Winnipeg MB R3E 0W2

CONTACT INFORMATION:
Telephone: 204-789-3499
Fax: 204-272-3169

E-Mail: admissions@med.umanitoba.ca
Website: http://umanitoba.ca/faculties/health_sciences/medicine/

GENERAL INFORMATION:

The University of Manitoba was founded in 1877. The University is a key part of the healthcare system in Western Canada and is involved with multiple national and international initiatives. The overall curriculum is based on the CanMeds-Family Medicine competency framework.

The mission of the University of Manitoba is to develop, deliver, and evaluate high quality educational programs for the benefit of undergraduate and postgraduate students. The school seeks to conduct research and disseminate information to health professions. The institution offers a bilingual education stream that enables providers to develop a solid grounding in both English and French.

The school does offer a summer preparatory program as well as an MD/PhD program for interested students.

On Campus Housing is available.

PREREQUISITES:

A baccalaureate degree of either three of four years of study is required upon admission.

AP/IB: Accepted with high exam scores

Required Courses (laboratory work with science coursework is expected):

Biochemistry – 1 year	Humanities – 1 year	Social Sciences – 1 year

The biochemistry course must be completed with a minimum grade of a C and be equivalent to the Biochemistry course taught at the University of Manitoba. Most students will have taken courses in Biology, Physical Chemistry, Mathematics, Physics, English, French, and Organic Chemistry. Eighteen hours in the humanities and social sciences is required.

Testing of Language Proficiency: Yes
MCAT® Required: Yes
AMRCB® transcript: Send via direct mail

MCAT®

MCAT Required: Yes

Average MCAT: >30

Average MCAT Bio: 10.4
Average MCAT Phys: 10.0
Average MCAT Verbal: 10.0
Average MCAT Essay: Q

MCAT minimum: 7/7/7/M

GPA:

4.14: GPA (overall on 4.5 scale)
3.3: GPA (minimum on 4.5 scale)

Combined Programs:

MD/BSc Med, MD/PhD

CURRICULUM:

Basic Sciences:

The basic science education is structured around six blocks of primary education with the development of clinical skills throughout the first two years.

Basic Sciences

Year 1	Year 2
Block 1: Structure, Function, and Disease Mechanisms Population Health and Medicine	Block 4: Endocrine and Metabolism Kidney Reproduction
Block 2: Human Development	Block 5: Musculoskeletal Ophthalmology Neurosciences
Block 3: Cardiovascular Ear, Nose, and Throat Respiratory Structure, Function, and Disease Mechanisms	Block 6: Blood and Lymph Gastrointestinal Dermatology
Clinical Skills	Clinical Skills
Problem Solving	Problem Solving
Medical Ethics and Humanities	Medical Ethics and Humanities
Laboratory Medicine	Laboratory Medicine
Survival Tactics	Survival Tactics

Clinical Sciences:

The clinical education begins with a five-week Introduction to Clerkship program which prepares students for the clerkship rotations.

Clinical Skills

Required Clerkships	Electives and Selectives
Internal Medicine – 6 weeks Surgery – 6 weeks Psychiatry – 6 weeks Pediatrics – 6 weeks OB/GYN – 6 weeks Family/Community Medicine – 6 weeks Multi-Specialty Rotation – 6 weeks • Emergency Medicine • Anesthesia • Otolaryngology • Ophthalmology • Community Health	Selectives Surgery – 6 weeks Medicine and Surgery – 6 weeks Electives Fourth Year Electives – 21 weeks

Thesis/Research Required: Optional
Community Service Requirements: Optional

TUITION: All currency listings are in Canadian Dollars (CAD)

Canadian Residents: $7,912
Compulsory Fees: $1,023

Application Fee: $90

Acceptance Deposit: $500 (non-refundable) – applied toward tuition

INTERVIEW:

Interviews: Multiple Mini Interviews (MMI) take place in February and March each year. A total of 278 applicants were interviewed in 2014. Of the applicants, 250 were from Manitoba and 28 applicants were from other areas of Canada. For applicants to the bilingual stream, a portion of the interview will be in French as well as English. A separate Aboriginal Interview Panel is in place for Aboriginal Applicants.

Acceptance Notification: E-mailed in May and June each year.

SELECTION FACTORS:

Accepted students usually have a grade point average between 3.9-4.5 on the 4.5 grading scale. The non-Science GPA is evaluated as well. An overall composite score (Adjusted GPA) is determined for each applicant which is used in the selection process. The MCAT® is used and individual sub-test scores must not be less than 7 and the writing score must not be less than an M for applicants from Manitoba. Accepted applicants generally have a sub-test sores great than 10 in all areas. Applicants are assigned an operative MCAT® score which is generated from the individual sub-test scores. Applicants that are not residents of Manitoba should not have a GPA lower than 3.94 or MCAT® scores on any subject lower than 10.75 in order to be considered.

The Admissions Committee expects applicants to have involvement with, and connection to, rural communities in Canada. Applications from students from rural areas are weighted to favor these applicants. Volunteer and work experiences are vital to the growth of students. Applicants are sought that will make a positive contribution to their profession and the public. Students are sought that have a sense of responsibility, maturity, and social skills. Applicants are expected to be successful academically as well. The Admissions Committee evaluates an applicant's extracurricular activities and exposure to the medical profession. Letters of recommendation are used to identify the suitability of applicants.

Priority is given to residents of Manitoba. Applicants who have been in the Canadian Forces for a minimum of two-years are considered in the pool of Manitoba applicants regardless of their residency. Aboriginal students are interviewed by a separate Admissions Committee but still must meet minimum eligibility requirements. Applicants with a PhD and academic appointment in a research or professional stream, and those with peer-reviewed publications are given additional consideration.

Table 1: University of Manitoba Applicant Match Statistics^*

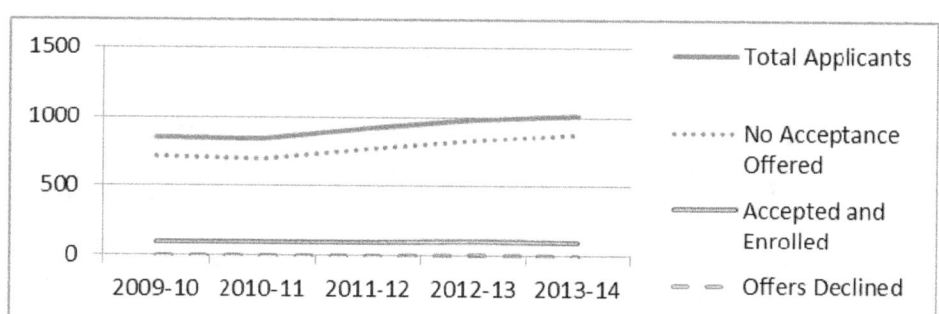

^ Success rate is defined as the percentage of applicants receiving at least one offer of admission regardless of acceptance
* Includes Canadian citizens/landed immigrants who were living outside Canada at time of application
Source: Admission Requirements of Canadian Faculties of Medicine

Table 2: University of Manitoba Applicant Selection Success

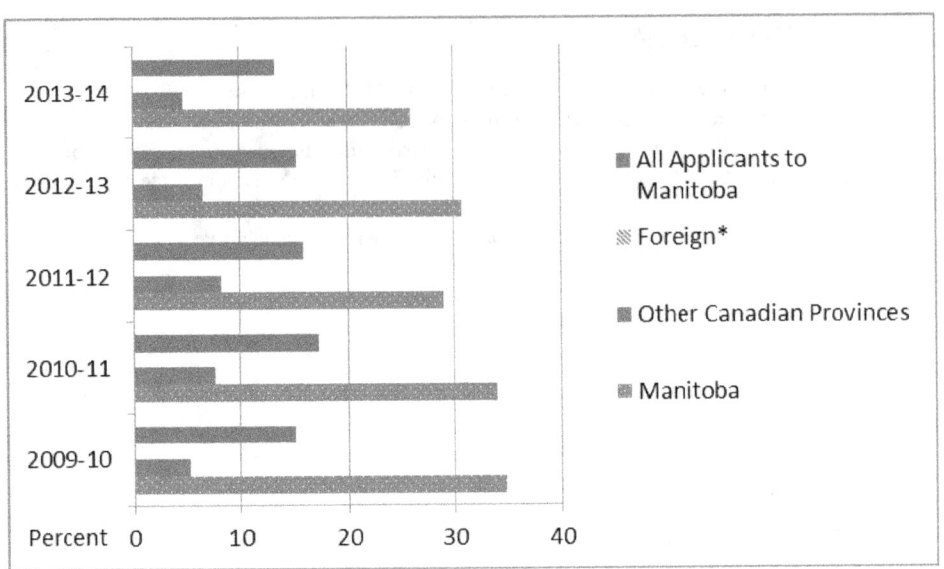

Source: Admission Requirements of Canadian Faculties of Medicine

Newfoundland

Memorial University of Newfoundland, Faculty of Medicine

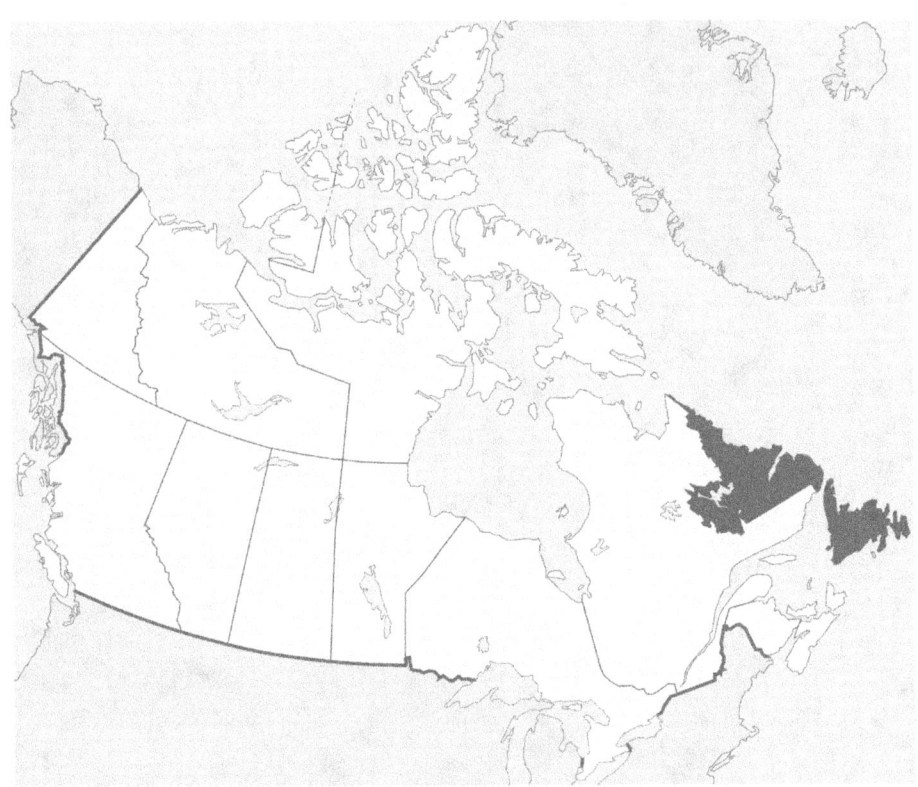

Memorial University of Newfoundland, Faculty of Medicine

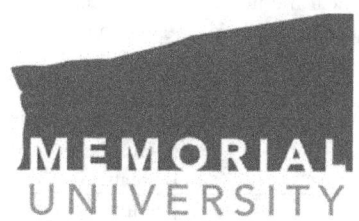

QUICK FACTS

POSITIONS:
80: Total
60: Newfoundland/Labrador
10: New Brunswick
4: Prince Edward Island
1: Yukon
4: Out-of-Province
3: Aboriginal

Male/Female %: 48/52

UNIVERSITY:
Type: Public

APPLICATIONS:
Accept Non-Canadians: Yes
Transfers: Yes
Deferred Admissions: Yes

Primary Application: CaRMS

Secondary Application: No

Early Decision: No

CURRICULUM:
Length: 4-years
Language: English

Dr. James Rourke - Dean, Faculty of Medicine

CAMPUS:
Committee on Admissions
Admissions Office, Faculty of Medicine
Memorial University of Newfoundland
Health Sciences Centre Room 1751
St. John's NL A1B 3V6

CONTACT INFORMATION:
Telephone: 1-855-633-9800 or 709-777-6615
Fax: 709-777-8422

E-Mail: admissions@carms.ca
Website: http://www.med.mun.ca/admissions

GENERAL INFORMATION:

Memorial University of Newfoundland was initially founded in 1925 becoming a full university in 1949. The Faculty of Medicine was founded in 1968 with the first students starting in 1969. The university recently went through an expansion in 2013 with the addition of the Craig L. Dobbin Genetics Research Centre and additional space was added for the medical education center. This expansion allowed Memorial University to increase the class size from 60 to 80 students each year.

The mission of the university is to enhance the health of people by educating physicians and health scientists, by conducting research in clinical and basic medical sciences and applied health sciences, and by promoting the skills and attitudes of lifelong learning. Students are able to take either the Canadian or United States licensing examinations through the curriculum.

The school does offer a summer, preparatory program for interested students. Dual degree programs are available to qualified students.

Campus Housing is available for single and married students.

PREREQUISITES:

A Bachelor's degree and six credit hours in English are required at the time of admission. In exceptional circumstances an application may be considered when a Bachelor's degree will not be held at time of admission.

Required Courses: English – 6 credit hours

No absolute prerequisites are in place other than English, although a solid science background is expected.

Testing of Language Proficiency: No
MCAT® Required: Yes
AMRCB® transcript: submitted electronically directly through CaRMS

MCAT®

MCAT Required: Yes

Average MCAT: 30

Average MCAT Bio: 10.0
Average MCAT Phys: 9.0
Average MCAT Verbal:: 9.0
Average MCAT Essay: O

GPA:

3.8: GPA (overall)

Combined Programs:

MD/MSC, MD/PhD

CURRICULUM:

Basic Sciences:

The first two years are divided into three phases. Phase 1 focuses on the healthy person and wellness. Phase 2 emphasizes acute reversible or modifiable health issues, whereas Phase 3 continues with an emphasis on chronic illness. Clinical medicine is introduced during the basic science instruction. Seminars, small-group learning, lectures, laboratories, and open discussions are all utilized.

Basic Sciences

Phase 1	Phase 2	Phase 3
The Healthy Person	The Patient: Acute or Episodic Health Problems	The Patient: Chronic Conditions
Clinical Skills I	Clinical Skills II	Clinical Skills III
Special Projects I	Special Projects II	Special Projects III
Community Engagement I	Community Engagement II	

Clinical Sciences:

Training takes place at Dr. Charles A. Jameway Clinic Health Centre, Grace General Hospital, St. Clare's Mercy Hospital, University General Hospital, Waterford Hospital, and other non-affiliated hospitals.

Clinical Skills

Required Clerkships	Electives and Selectives
Internal Medicine – 8 weeks Surgery – 8 weeks Psychiatry – 8 weeks Pediatrics – 8 weeks OB/GYN – 8 weeks Rural Family Medicine – 4 weeks	Electives – 20 weeks Advanced Practice Integration

Thesis/Research Required: Optional - students are able to initiate Basic Science research if desired
Community Service Requirements: Yes – visits to community-based clinics and hospitals

TUITION: All currency listings are in Canadian Dollars (CAD)

Canadian Residents: $6,250   International/Visa Students: $30,000
Compulsory Fees: $1,220

Application Fee: $75 (plus $150 CaRMS application)

CaRMS Application: https://mun.e-carms.ca/medusa-web/login
Acceptance Deposit: $200 (non-refundable) – applied toward tuition

INTERVIEW:

Interviews take place in November for the entering class the following year. For 2014, a total of 229 applicants were interviewed for the 80 spots. Of the 229 applicants interviewed, 125 residents were from Newfoundland and Labrador and 104 were from other Canadian provinces. A combination of traditional interviews and Multiple-Mini interviews are utilized.

Acceptance Notification: Mailed via priority mail between February and May each year

SELECTION FACTORS:

The Admissions Committee seeks to identify the best qualified students. Only Canadian residents or visa students are eligible to apply for consideration, and the majority of positions are reserved for residents of Newfoundland and Labrador. Of the 80 available positions, three are available to Aboriginal students who are residents of Newfoundland and Labrador.

Other than the required prerequisite coursework, students are expected to have overall solid and well-rounded applications with high academic standards expected. The Admissions Committee looks favorably on work related experience and prior exposure to the healthcare field in a variety of settings. An applicant's essay, letters of recommendation, exposure to the medical profession, and extracurricular activities are considered as well. Students are sought who demonstrate humanistic qualities and attitudes that are necessary for physicians. An applicant's personal circumstances and potential disadvantaging factors are also considered. The interview is a significant factor in the selection process. One academic reference letter is preferred.

The MCAT® is required of all applicants with an average score of those accepted at a 10 in each category and a Q on the writing section. Science and non-Science GPA's are both considered, with the average GPA of accepted students at 3.7. No minimum cumulative GPA or MCAT® scores exist however.

Table 1: Memorial University Applicant Selection Success^*

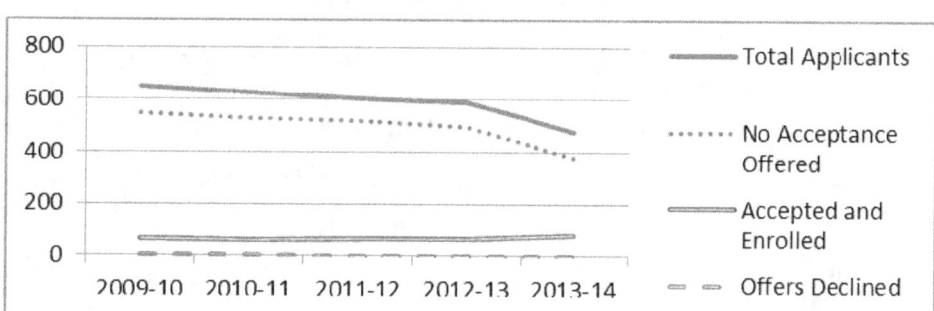

^ Success rate is defined as the percentage of applicants receiving at least one offer of admission regardless of acceptance
* Includes Canadian citizens/landed immigrants who were living outside Canada at time of application
Source: Admission Requirements of Canadian Faculties of Medicine

Table 2: Memorial University Applicant Match Statistics

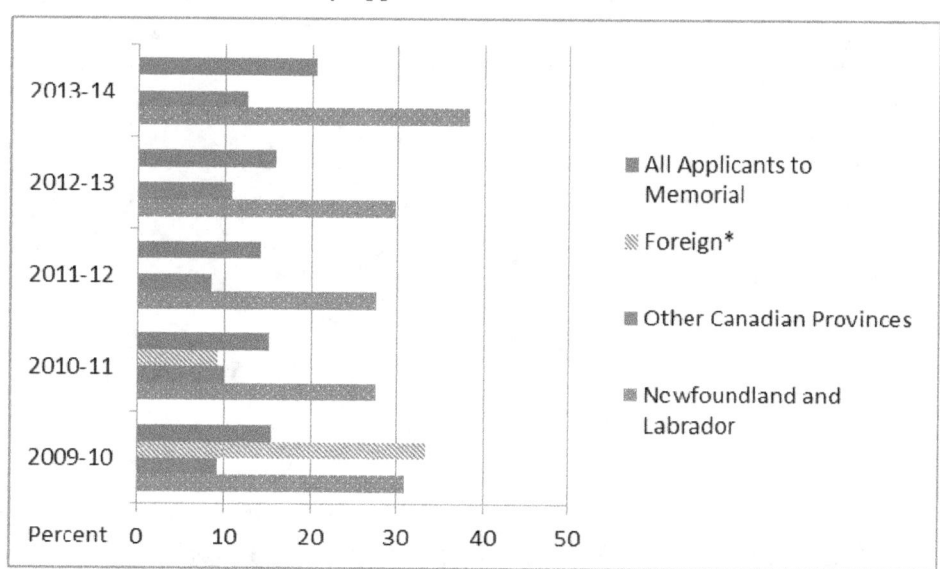

Source: Admission Requirements of Canadian Faculties of Medicine

Nova Scotia

Dalhousie University, Faculty of Medicine

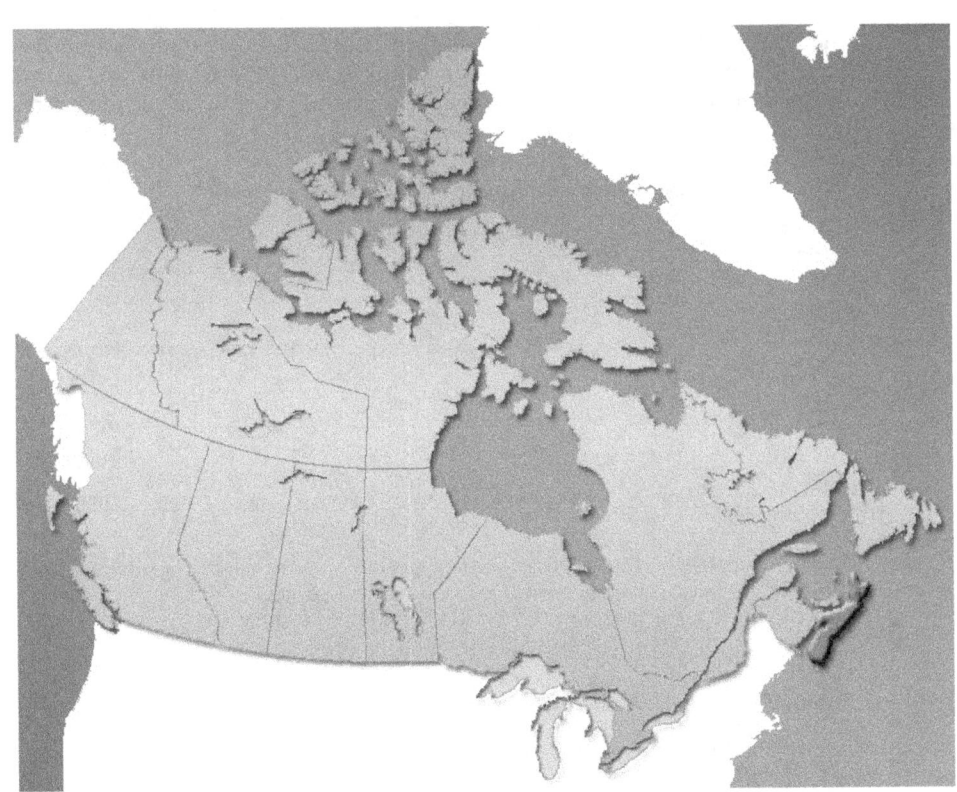

Dalhousie University, Faculty of Medicine

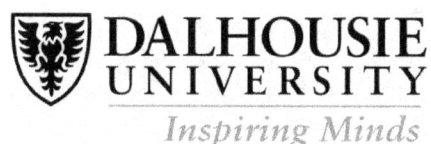

QUICK FACTS

POSITIONS:
109: Total
100: Maritime Resident
9: Out-of-province
1: Seat for Dental Student to specialize in maxillofacial surgery
69: Seats in Halifax Campus
30: Seats in St John Campus

Average age of 1st year: 24
Male/Female %: 44/56

UNIVERSITY:
Type: Public

APPLICATIONS:
Accept Non-Canadians: Yes
Transfers: No
Deferred Admissions: Yes

Primary Application:
Electronic - School Specific

Secondary Application: Yes

Early Decision: No

CURRICULUM:
Length: 4-years
Language: English

Dr. Thomas J. Marrie - Dean, Faculty of Medicine

CAMPUS:
Admissions & Student Affairs
Dalhousie University
Clinical Research Centre
5849 University Avenue
PO Box 15000
Halifax, NS B3H 4R2

CONTACT INFORMATION:
Telephone: 902-494-1874
Fax: 902-494-6369

E-Mail: medicine.admissions@dal.ca
Website: http://admissions.medicine.dal.ca/

GENERAL INFORMATION:

Dalhousie University Faculty of Medicine was founded in 1868. The medical school is responsible to New Brunswick, Nova Scotia, and Prince Edward Island. The student body is divided between the St. John campus and the Halifax campus. Approximately 78 students are assigned to the Halifax campus with the remaining assigned to the St. John campus. Combined degree programs are available for qualified students.

The mission of the school is to strive to benefit society through equal commitment to exemplary patient care, education, and the discovery and advancement of knowledge. The school aims to create and maintain a learning and research environment of national and international stature which enables graduates to serve the health needs of the Maritime Provinces and Canada. The school aims to provide a basic education that would permit a graduate to enter any branch of postgraduate training. The curriculum was recently updated drawing on best practices, student input, and current educational models.

Campus Housing is available

PREREQUISITES:

A Bachelor's degree is required at the time of admission. Students must have had a full course load of five full classes each year over the two most recent years of study in order to be eligible to apply. Summer classes do not count toward course load requirements.

No absolute prerequisites are in place, although a solid science background is expected. Students are expected to have pursued diverse and challenging topics and to have had a natural progression in their degree completion.

Testing of Language Proficiency: No
MCAT® Required: Yes
AMRCB® transcript: Submit via mail directly to the school.

<u>MCAT®</u>

MCAT Required: Yes

Average MCAT: 31

Average MCAT Bio: 10.0
Average MCAT Phys: 10.0
Average MCAT Verbal: 11.37
Average MCAT Essay: O

<u>GPA:</u>

3.8: GPA (overall)
3.3: GPA (minimum)

3.3: Maritime Resident
minimum GPA

3.7: Non-Maritime Resident
minimum GPA

<u>Combined Programs:</u>

MD/MSc, MD/PhD

CURRICULUM:

Basic Sciences:

The curriculum uses a progressive Case-Oriented Problem-Simulated (COPS) curriculum. Group learning, clinical interaction with patients and contextual learning are all used. Students are organized into small groups and have patient contact through Patient-Doctor sessions.

Basic Sciences

Year 1	Year 2
Foundations of Medicine	Neurosciences (Ventral Nervous System and Special senses)
Host Defense (Hematology, Infection, Immunity and Inflammation)	Metabolism II (Cardiovascular, Respiratory and Renal)
Metabolism (Gastroenterology, Endocrinology, Nutrition, and Oral Medicine)	Musculoskeletal & Dermatology
Human Development	Integration
Professional Competencies I	Professional Competencies II
Skilled Clinician Program	Skilled Clinician Program
Research in Medicine	Research in Medicine
Electives	Electives

Clinical Sciences:

The clerkships are organized into two phases, both which begin with a four week introduction. Instruction occurs at a Pediatric hospital, OB/GYN Hospital, two large tertiary care hospitals, a Psychiatric hospital, community clinics, and a rehabilitation hospital.

Clinical Skills

Required Clerkships	Electives and Selectives

Medicine – 12 weeks
Surgery – 9 weeks
Psychiatry – 6 weeks
Pediatrics – 6 weeks
OB/GYN – 6 weeks
Family Medicine – 6 weeks
Emergency Medicine – 3 weeks
	Third Year Electives – 18 weeks
	
	Fourth Year Electives – 18 weeks
	   • General Electives – 12 weeks
	   • Community Based – 3 weeks
	   • Interdisciplinary – 3 weeks

Thesis/Research Required: Optional
Community Service Requirements: Optional

TUITION: All currency listings are in Canadian Dollars (CAD)

Canadian Residents: $17,430   Visa Students: $25,878   Foreign Students: $75,000
Compulsory Fees: $1,101

Visa students (International / US students) pay a differential fee of $4,224.00/term (2 terms) on top of the regular tuition fees.

The application process involves two-steps. Step one is due mid-August and this be must be submitted prior to Step 2 which is due by September 1st.

Application Fee: $70
Acceptance Deposit: $500 (non-refundable) – applied toward tuition

INTERVIEW:

Multiple-Mini interviews are utilized in the interview process for all students. All Maritime residents who meet the minimum requirements for admission will be extended an interview. In 2014, a total of 351 students were interviewed of which 292 were Maritime residents and 59 were non-Maritime residents.

Acceptance Notification: Mailed in March each year

SELECTION FACTORS:

Applicants considered include Canadian citizens and permanent residents, those with a Canadian visa, and international students. For the 109 positions each year, nearly 100 are filled by Maritime resident of Nova Scotia, New Brunswick, and Prince Edward Island. The remaining positions are open to international applications. Of those accepted from the Maritime regions, 69 will be assigned to the campus in Halifax and 30 will be assigned to the St. John Campus. One position is available to a dental student who plans to specialize in oral maxillofacial surgery after completing medical school.

The Admissions Committee considers the letters of recommendation, MCAT® scores, essays, the non-science GPA, extracurricular activities, and exposure to the medical profession. Students receive an overall score based on their GPA, MCAT®, essay, and interview score. Students are sought who will be professional, contribute to the community, are lifelong learners, and who will become skilled clinicians. No quotas are in place for specific demographic factors. Students are not likely to be selected if they have an academic record that shows repeated or failed classes. The interview plays an important part of the selection process. Non-Maritime applicants are expected to have outstanding qualifications in order to be considered

The average MCAT® score of those accepted to the program is an overall score of 29 with a writing score of a Q. The minimum GPA to be considered for an interviewed is 3.3 with the average GPA of accepted students at 3.8 overall. The average GPA of accepted students from the Maritime provinces is 3.3 and 3.7 for non-Maritime residents.

Table 1: Dalhousie University Applicant Match Statistics^*

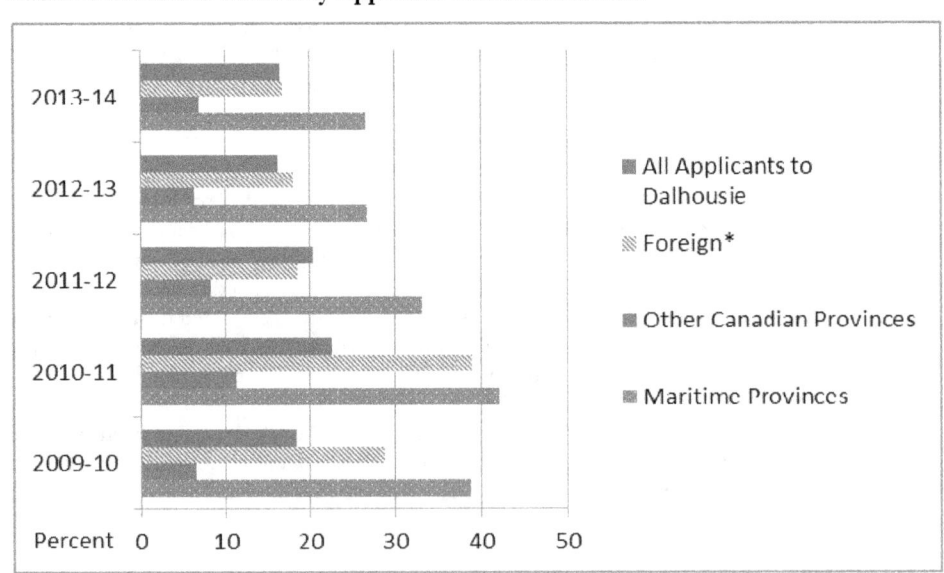

^ Success rate is defined as the percentage of applicants receiving at least one offer of admission regardless of acceptance
* Includes Canadian citizens/landed immigrants who were living outside Canada at time of application
Source: Admission Requirements of Canadian Faculties of Medicine

Table 2: Dalhousie University Applicant Selection Success

Source: Admission Requirements of Canadian Faculties of Medicine

Ontario

McMaster University, Michael G. DeGroote School of Medicine

Northern Ontario School of Medicine

University of Ottawa, Faculty of Medicine

Queen's University, School of Medicine

University of Toronto, Faculty of Medicine

Western University, Schulich School of Medicine and Dentistry

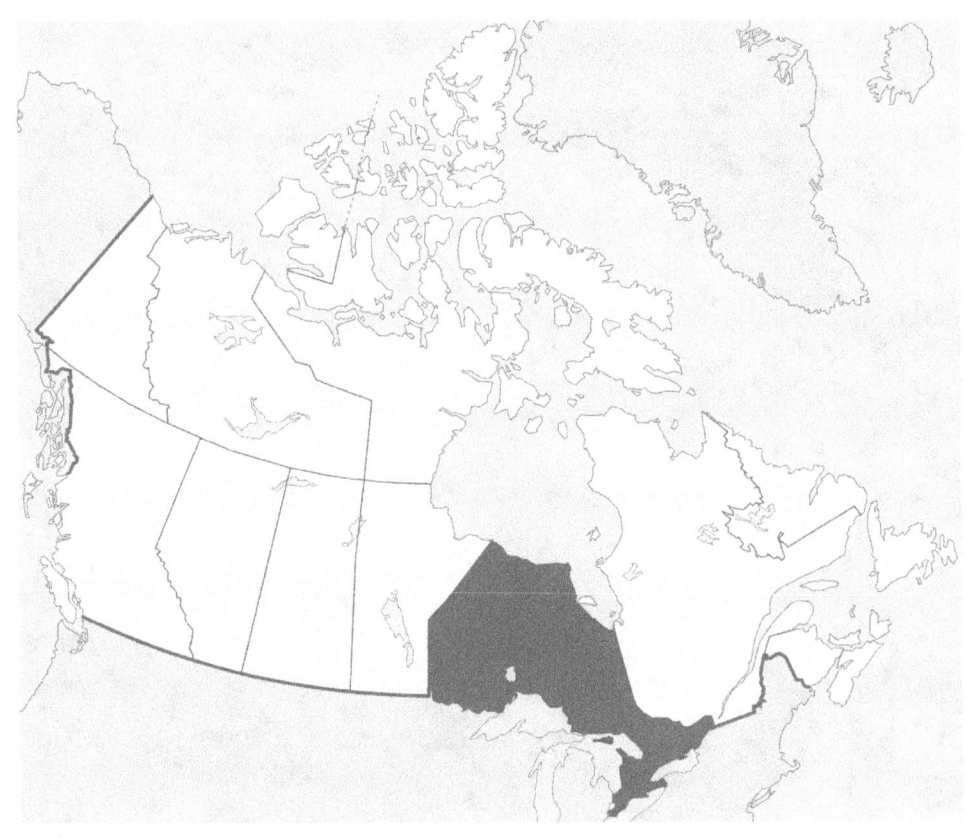

McMaster University, Michael G. DeGroote School of Medicine

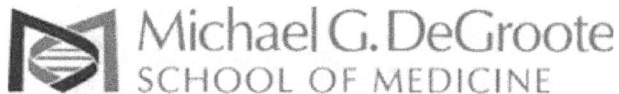

Dr. John Kelton - Dean & Vice-President

CAMPUS:
McMaster University MD Admissions
1280 Main Street West MDCL-3104
Hamilton ON L8S 4K1

CONTACT INFORMATION:
Telephone: 905-525-9140 (ext. 22235)
Fax: 905-546-0349

E-Mail: mdadmit@mcmaster.ca
Website: http://www.fhs.mcmaster.ca/mdprog

GENERAL INFORMATION:

McMaster University School of Medicine was founded in 1965 and renamed the Michael G. DeGroote School of Medicine in 2004. McMaster University operates three separate campuses. The main campus is the Hamilton Campus which houses 147 students from each class. Twenty-eight positions are available at the Waterloo Regional Campus which began in 2007 in Kitchener; and twenty-eight positions are at the Niagara Regional Campus in St. Catherine's which was founded in 2008. Students are able to specify their location of preference and do so at the time of interview. The curriculum at all three campuses is identical.

The mission of the school is to advance health through learning and discovery. The school strives to develop the personal attributes and personal characteristics and attitudes that are compatible with effective health care, the development of clinical and communication skills, and the development of lifelong learners. The curriculum allows for flexibility to allow for varying backgrounds and career goals and uses problem-based educational methods with the central focus of the program on tutorial education. Students are taught to develop critical thinking skills, clinical skills, and self-directed learning skills.

A combined MD/PhD program is available for interested students.

Campus Housing is available.

PREREQUISITES:

A minimum of three years of university credit is required. No specific prerequisite courses are required prior to admission. An adequate background in the sciences is expected.

Testing of Language Proficiency: Yes
The MCAT® is required, but only the verbal reasoning score is used in selection
AMRCB® transcripts are mailed directly to OMSAS for inclusion in the application

MCAT®

MCAT Required: Yes

Average MCAT-VR:
10.86 (only VR Considered)

MCAT/VR minimum: 6

GPA:

3.83: GPA (overall)
3.0: GPA (minimum)

Combined Programs:

MD/PhD

CURRICULUM:

Basic Sciences:

The school utilizes problem-based learning which began originally in 1969 at McMaster University. The curriculum is entitled the COMPASS curriculum and focuses on the mastery of fundamental concepts of medicine. The pre-clerkship, basic science years are divided into five Medical Foundation blocks and runs throughout the three years of the program.

Basic Sciences

Medical Foundation 1	Medical Foundation 2	Medical Foundation 3	Medical Foundation 4	Medical Foundation 5
Oxygen Supply – Respiratory, Hematologic, and Cardiovascular	Homeostasis – GI, Endocrine System, and Nutrition	Homeostasis – Renal, Reproduction, and Pregnancy	Host Defense - Immunology, Infectious Disease, Neoplasia	Movement - Locomotor System, Nervous System, and Behavior
Professional Competencies				

Clinical Sciences:

The clinical clerkships are conducted at teaching hospitals in Hamilton; in community hospitals, including those in St. Catharines, Guelph, Brantford, Burlington, Niagara Falls and the Kitchener-Waterloo region; and in association with the Northwest Ontario Medical Program.

Clinical Sciences

Variable duration during the three year curriculum	
Medicine Surgery Pediatrics OB / GYN Family Medicine Psychiatry Anesthesia Emergency Medicine Geriatrics	Electives (1/2 must be in clinical electives)

Thesis/Research Required: Optional
Community Service Requirements: Optional

TUITION: All currency listings are in Canadian Dollars (CAD)

Canadian Residents: $26,416   Visa Students: $95,871   Foreign Students: $95,000
Compulsory Fees: $871

Application Fee: OMSAS $210, Secondary Application Fee $115
Acceptance Deposit: $1,000 (non-refundable) – applied toward tuition

INTERVIEW:

Interviews: Multiple Mini Interviews (MMI) take place in March and April each year. A total of 550 applicants were interviewed in 2014, of which one was from outside of Canada. Students list their preference of campus locations at the time of interview. Offers of admission are binding to the assigned campus. Aboriginal applicants will be interviewed by a separate panel.

Acceptance Notification in the spring each year.

SELECTION FACTORS:

The MCAT® is required for admission, but only the Verbal Reasoning section is used. A minimum score of 6 is required on the Verbal Reasoning section, and scoring on the other sections are not considered. For the new MCAT®, a minimum score of 123 is required on the Critical Analysis and Reasoning Section. Only the most recent MCAT® score will be considered. Invitations for interview are based on academic performance and assessment of the preparedness for a career in medicine and suitability for the program.

The Admissions Committee seeks to select students that have high academic standards, but also those that are able to demonstrate the characteristics deemed to be important for the study and practice of medicine. Desired characteristics include sensitivity to the emotional, psychological, and the physical aspects of patients; the ability to solve and detect problems; the ability to learn independently; and ability to function in a small group, and the ability to be sensitive to the needs of the community. Applicants are selected based on non-cognitive and the overall academic qualities of each applicant considered. Students are selected regardless of their geographical preference of campus location. Offers of admission are binding to the campus assigned. Applicants are selected that will have the flexibility and capacity to practice broadly in the field of medicine.

Applicant statistics are not reported currently for medical schools located in Ontario.

Northern Ontario School of Medicine

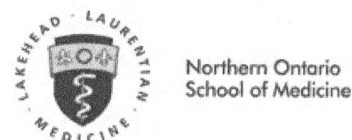

Northern Ontario
School of Medicine

QUICK FACTS

POSITIONS:
64: Total
62: General
2: Aboriginal

Average age of 1st year: 25
Male/Female %: 41/59

UNIVERSITY:
Type: Public

APPLICATIONS:
Accept Non-Canadians: No
Transfers: No
Deferred Admissions: Yes

Primary Application:
OMSAS

Secondary Application: Yes

Early Decision: No

CURRICULUM:
Length: 4-years
Language: English

Dr. Roger Strasser - Founding Dean

CAMPUS:
Office of Admissions
Northern Ontario School of Medicine
955 Oliver Road MS 2003,
Thunder Bay ON P7B 5E1

CONTACT INFORMATION:
Telephone: 807-766-7463 or 1-800-461-8777
Fax: 807-766-7368

E-Mail: admissions@nosm.ca
Website: http://www.nosm.ca

GENERAL INFORMATION:

The Northern Ontario School of Medicine was founded in 2005 and was the first new school in Canada in the 21st century. The school has two campuses, The Lakehead (West) Campus and the Laurentian (East) Campus. The Lakehead Campus instructs 28 students with the Laurentian campus instructing 36 students. Students are able to select a preference of campus locations but no guarantee is in place regarding assignment. Students will be asked their preference of location if invited for an interview.

The mission of the school is to be committed to the education of high quality physicians and health professionals, and to gain international recognition as a leader in distributed, community-engaged, learning-centered education and research. The curriculum is based on real-life, patient-centered, and case-based learning. The school operates several educational programs including a physician assistant program and post-graduate programs.

Campus Housing is available.

PREREQUISITES:

A bachelorette degree or equivalent is required prior to admission. An exception is made for students who are 25 years or older as they may apply with a three-year degree. No specific prerequisites are in place, although a broad education in the sciences, humanities, and social sciences are expected.

All science majors should have completed at a minimum:

Arts – 2 courses   Social Sciences – 2 courses   Humanities – 2 courses
Science Courses in their specific degree program – 2 courses

Testing of Language Proficiency: Yes
MCAT® required: No
AMRCB® transcripts are mailed directly to OMSAS for inclusion in the application

MCAT®

MCAT Required: No

Average MCAT: NA

GPA:

3.83: GPA (overall)
3.0: GPA (minimum)

Combined Programs:

None

CURRICULUM:

Basic Sciences:

The Basic Science education utilizes small and large group teaching, community-based experiences, and practical and lab teaching. Students complete a 4-week community-based clinical experience in an Aboriginal community at the end of year one and two small community placements in year two.

Basic Sciences	
Phase 1	
Year 1	**Year 2**
Review and Introduction	Reproductive System
Gastrointestinal System	Renal System
Cardiovascular/Respiratory Systems	Haematology/Immunology
Central Nervous System / Peripheral Nervous System	Mental Health and Cognitive Impairment
Musculoskeletal System	End of Life Issues
Endocrine System	

Clinical Sciences:

Rotations occurs in medium-sized Northern Ontario communities.

Clinical Sciences – Year 3
Phase 2
Comprehensive Community Clerkship – 8 months

Clinical Rotations – Year 4	
Phase 3	
Surgery – 4 weeks Internal Medicine – 4 weeks Children's Health – 4 weeks Women's Health – 4 weeks Mental Health – 4 weeks Emergency Medicine – 4 weeks Family Medicine – 4 weeks	Electives – 12 weeks

Thesis/Research Required: Optional
Community Service Requirements: Required

TUITION: All currency listings are in Canadian Dollars (CAD)

Canadian Residents: $21,845
Compulsory Fees: $798 Lakehead (West Campus), $1,029 Laurentian (East) Campus

Application Fee: OMSAS $210, Secondary Application $85

Applicants complete the undergraduate application first, followed by a secondary application.
Acceptance Deposit: $1,000 (non-refundable) – applied toward tuition

INTERVIEW:

Interviews: Take place in March each year. A total of 321 applicants were interviewed in 2014 from a pool of 2,130 applicants. A Mini-Interview format is utilized.

Acceptance Notification: Mailed in May each year.

SELECTION FACTORS:

Only Canadian citizens and permanent residents are eligible to apply and the Admissions Committee aims to maximize the recruitment of students from Northern Ontario and those with the interest and aptitude to practice in rural and remote communities. A minimum grade point average of 3.0 on a 4.0 scale is required for consideration, although the average GPA of accepted applicants was 3.83 in 2014. The MCAT® is not required. A four-year undergraduate degree is required, except for applicants who are 25 years or older who may apply with a three-year degree. Students with a graduate degree are given additional credit in the application process. Applications are screened based on the GPA, the application questionnaire and autobiographical sketch, and a context score derived from the applicant's current and past geographical residence.

The Admissions Committee selects students based on academic and autobiographical information. Applicants are assigned an overall score based on their academic success, school submission questions, place of residence, as well as other submitted information. Applicants are invited to interview based on their overall application score. Students are sought who have a genuine interest in fulfilling and upholding the values of the institution. The Admissions Committee looks favorably on volunteer work, cross-cultural experiences, and extra-curricular activities. The interview is an important part of the selection process. The Admissions Committee seeks to identify those with interpersonal skills and appropriate decision-making capacities. Applicants are selected that will thrive in rural and northern communities. Selection favors Aboriginal applicants, Francophone applicants, and those from rural and remote areas of Northern Ontario and Canada. Aboriginal applicants must still meet minimum application requirements.

Applicant statistics are not reported currently for medical schools located in Ontario.

University of Ottawa, Faculty of Medicine

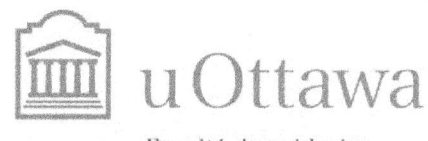

Faculté de médecine
Faculty of Medicine

QUICK FACTS

POSITIONS:
164: Total
8: Above Quota Positions
7: Aboriginal
4: MD/PhD Program

Average age of 1st year: 24
Male/Female %: 44/56

UNIVERSITY:
Type: Public

APPLICATIONS:
Accept Non-Canadians: No
Transfers: Yes
Deferred Admissions: Yes

Primary Application:
OMSAS

Secondary Application: Yes

Early Decision: No

CURRICULUM:
Length: 4-years
Language: English and
French

Dr. Jacques Bradwejn - Dean, Faculty of Medicine

CAMPUS:
University of Ottawa
Admissions - Faculty of Medicine
University of Ottawa,
451 Smyth Road Room 2044
Ottawa ON K1H 8M5

CONTACT INFORMATION:
Telephone: 613-562-5409
Fax: 613-562-5605

E-Mail: admissmd@uottawa.ca
Website: http://www.medicine.uottawa.ca

GENERAL INFORMATION:

The University of Ottawa Faculty of Medicine was founded in 1945. The school emphasizes self-directed learning with students acquiring the knowledge, skills, and attitudes needed to understand and apply effective medicine. Training is designed to foster compassion, communication skills, trust, patient advocacy, and ethical and professional conduct.

The mission of the school is to develop society's leaders who improve the health of Canadians and communities worldwide. This is done through education, patient care, research, and technology in an inclusive environment. The school emphasizes health promotion and disease prevention and strives to be responsive to the changes in society and the healthcare system. The educational process is conducted in both French and English.

In addition to the 164 students admitted each year, up to eight above quota positions are available through the Consortium national de formation en sante. An MD/PhD program is available to interested students.

On campus housing is available.

PREREQUISITES:

A minimum of three years of full-time study leading to a Bachelor's degree is required.

Required Courses (laboratory work with science coursework is expected):

General Chemistry – 1 year   Biochemistry – 1 year   Organic Chemistry – 1 year
Biology or Zoology – 1 year   Humanities/Social Sciences – 2 years

Students are encouraged to have had a broad exposure to biology, the physical sciences, the arts, humanities, and social sciences. Several options are accepted as methods of completing the biochemistry requirement. Applicants are expected to be computer literate.

Testing of Language Proficiency: If needed on an individual basis.
MCAT® required: No
AMRCB® transcripts are mailed directly to OMSAS for inclusion in the application

<u>MCAT®</u>

MCAT Required: No

Average MCAT: NA

<u>GPA:</u>

3.91: GPA (overall)
3.5: GPA (minimum)

<u>Combined Programs:</u>

MD/PhD

<u>CURRICULUM:</u>

<u>Basic Sciences:</u>

The Basic Sciences are taught in a multi-disciplinary fashion with emphasis on the context of clinical problems. Seminars and lectures are utilized. The program integrates the Basic Sciences and Clinical Sciences throughout the four years.

Basic Sciences

Years 1 and 2 – 68 weeks
Introduction to the Profession
Foundations Unit
Basic principles of molecular and cellular biology, genetics, immunology, microbiology, blood cells, and neoplasia
Unit I
Principles of hemostatic control of body systems, oxygen transport, and hemostasis
Unit II
Principles of embryology, anatomy, histology, physiology and pathophysiology of the endocrine systems, of the male and female reproductive systems, and of the gastrointestinal and hepatobiliary systems
Unit III
Principles of embryology, anatomy, histology, physiology and pathophysiology of the nervous system, including the eye and the ear, and psychiatric conditions.
Integrated Unit
Includes instruction on the pediatric patient, the geriatric patient, the management of pain, palliative care, pharmacotherapeutics, international health, complementary and alternative medicine, occupational and environmental health, and health systems
Physician Skills Development (Part 1)
Physician Skills Development (Part 2)

<u>Clinical Sciences:</u>

All students complete a month rotation in a rural setting.

Clinical Skills

Required Clerkships	Electives and Selectives
Internal Medicine – 6 weeks	Selectives – 6 weeks
Surgery – 6 weeks	Otolaryngology – 2 weeks
Psychiatry – 6 weeks	Ophthalmology – 2 weeks
Pediatrics – 6 weeks	Pediatrics – 2 weeks
OB/GYN – 6 weeks	
Family Medicine – 6 weeks	Fourth Year Electives – 18 weeks
Acute Care Medicine – 6 weeks	

Thesis/Research Required: Optional
Community Service Requirements: Required

<u>TUITION: All currency listings are in Canadian Dollars (CAD)</u>

Canadian Residents: $23,298
Compulsory Fees: $671

Application Fee: OMSAS $210, secondary application fee of $75
Acceptance Deposit: $1,000 (non-refundable) – applied toward tuition

INTERVIEW:

Interviews: Multiple Mini Interviews (MMI) take place in February and March each year. A total of 575 applicants were interviewed in 2014. Interviews will be conducted in the applicant's language of choice. A composite score is derived for each student from this process.

Acceptance Notification: Mailed beginning in May each year.

SELECTION FACTORS:

The Admissions Committee only accepts applicants from Canadian citizens and permanent residents, as well as applications from eligible children of alumni of the University of Ottawa who have completed their medical education at the Faculty of Medicine. Each year, the institution develops a weighted grade point average (WGPA) for the applicant pool and this number can vary each year. The WGPA is determined by the quality and quantity of the applications each year. The average entering GPA of accepted students was 3.91 in 2014. The MCAT® is not required for admission. An applicant's levels of difficulty during undergraduate study and the relevance to the study of medicine are considered.

The Admissions Committee seeks to identify applicants who have demonstrated academic success. Academic success is defined by the overall GPA of students and by comparison with other applicants. Students are encouraged to focus on their desired area of interest and no preference is given to any specific academic program. Students are encouraged to have had a broad exposure to biology, the physical sciences, the arts, humanities, and social sciences. The interview is an important aspect of the selection process and students are rated during the interview process.

Students who are identified as a francophone minority are admitted over and above the quota set by the Government of Ontario. Students who are proficient in French and English are given preference as well. The geographic status of each applicant is determined and this does play a role in the admissions process. The required GPA cut-off for aboriginal applicants is lower than other applicants.

Applicant statistics are not reported currently for medical schools located in Ontario.

Queen's University, School of Medicine

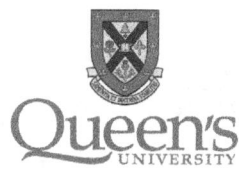

QUICK FACTS

POSITIONS:
100: Total
96: General
4:   Aboriginal

Male/Female %: 52/48

UNIVERSITY:
Type: Public

APPLICATIONS:
Accept Non-Canadians: No
Transfers: No
Deferred Admissions: Yes

Primary Application:
OMSAS

Secondary Application: Yes

Early Decision: No

CURRICULUM:
Length: 4-years
Language: English

Dr. Richard Reznick - Dean, Faculty of Health Sciences

CAMPUS:
Queen's University at Kingston
Admissions Officer
School of Medicine,
80 Barrie Street
Kingston ON K7L 3N6

CONTACT INFORMATION:
Telephone: 613-533-3307
Fax: 613-533-3190

E-Mail: queensmd@queensu.ca
Website: http://meds.queensu.ca/undergrad

GENERAL INFORMATION:

Queen's University Faculty of Health Sciences was founded in 1854. The University prides itself on the close, personal interaction between faculty and staff. The curriculum is designed to provide high levels of integration between the Basic and Clinical Sciences and to develop leaders in healthcare. The school embraces a spirit of innovation and inquiry in research and education.

The mission of the university is to advance the tradition of preparing excellent physicians. The goal of the university is to produce clinicians who have developed a wide understanding, knowledge, skills, and attitude to practice medicine. Although no formal programs are in place, students are able to enroll in multiple Master's and PhD programs within the University. Students obtain an extensive, hands-on clinical experience.

Campus housing and university rentals off-campus are available.

PREREQUISITES:

A minimum of three years of full-time university study is required, although students can apply prior to completion of the three years.

Although no specific coursework is required for admission, in general, students are expected to have at a minimum the following (laboratory work with science coursework is expected):

Biological Sciences – 1 year   Physical Sciences – 1 year   Humanities/Social Sciences – 1 year

Testing of Language Proficiency: No
MCAT® required: Yes
AMRCB® transcripts are mailed directly to OMSAS for inclusion in the application

MCAT®

MCAT Required: Yes

Average MCAT: 33

Average MCAT Bio: 11.0
Average MCAT Phys: 11.1
Average MCAT Verbal: 10.8
Average MCAT Essay: P

GPA:

3.7+: GPA (overall)

Combined Programs:

MD/MSc, MD/PhD

CURRICULUM:

Basic Sciences:

Problem-Based education, group discussions, lectures, laboratories, seminars, and computer-based instruction are utilized.

Basic Sciences

Year 1	Year 2
Scientific Foundation Courses • Normal Human Structure • Normal Human Function • Mechanism of Disease • Fundamentals of Therapeutics	Professional Foundation Courses • Critical Inquiry A and B • Professional Integration A and B
Clinical Foundation Courses • Family Medicine • Blood and Coagulation • Pediatrics and Genetics • Musculoskeletal • Principles of Geriatrics, Oncology, and Palliative Care	Clinical Foundation Courses • Circulatory and Respiratory • Endocrine and Renal • Gastroenterology and Surgery • Psychiatry • Genitourinary and Reproduction • Neurosciences • Skin and Special Senses
Professional Foundation Courses • Critical Appraisal, Research, and Learning • Professional Foundations 1A and 1B • Population and Global Health	Clinical and Communication Skills 2A and 2B
Clinical and Communications Skills 1A and 1B	

Clinical Sciences:

Clerkships are conducted at Hotel Dieu Hospital, Kingston General Hospital, Kingston Psychiatric Hospital, Ongwanada Hospital, Providence Continuing Care Centre, and St. Mary's of the Lake Hospital,

Clinical Sciences

Required Clerkships	Electives and Selectives
Medicine – 12 weeks Surgery – 8 weeks Psychiatry – 6 weeks Pediatrics – 6 weeks OB/GYN – 6 weeks Family Medicine – 4 weeks Emergency Medicine – 2 weeks Geriatrics – 2 weeks	Electives – 4 weeks Selectives – 12 weeks

Thesis/Research Required: Optional
Community Service Requirements: Optional

TUITION: All currency listings are in Canadian Dollars (CAD)

Canadian Residents: $23,445
Compulsory Fees: $1,110

Application Fee: OMSAS $210, secondary application fee of $100
Acceptance Deposit: $1,050 (non-refundable) – applied toward tuition

INTERVIEW:

Interviews: Take place in March each year. Students who advance through initial stages of GPA and MCAT® score requirements are invited for assessment of personal experiences and personal qualities.

Acceptance Notification: Mailed in May each year.

SELECTION FACTORS:

Only Canadian citizens, permanent residents, or children of alumni of Queen's University are considered for entry. Applicants are assessed overall on their cumulative grade point average which includes all coursework taken. For students who do not meet minimum requirements, the most recent two full-time years of student coursework will be considered. All students will have a cumulative GPA and most recent GPA over the last 2 years developed by the Admissions Committee. A minimum GPA is determined each year for applicants and this GPA can vary each year.   The MCAT® is required and the test must have been taken within 5 years. An MCAT® cut-off score is developed each year as well.

The Admissions Committee seeks students who have strong academic record and strong personal qualities. The Admissions Committee considers the essay, Science and Non-Science GPA's, extracurricular activities, and the letters of recommendation. A student's commitment, critical thinking ability, creativity, sensitivity, and ability to be self-directed are important for the Admissions Committee to recognize.   No specific undergraduate degree is favored. The interview is an important part of the selection process.

Applicant statistics are not reported currently for medical schools located in Ontario.

University of Toronto, Faculty of Medicine

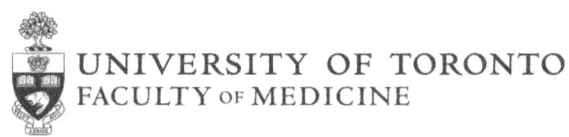

UNIVERSITY OF TORONTO
FACULTY ᴏꜰ MEDICINE

QUICK FACTS

POSITIONS:
259: Total
244: General
7: Foreign
8: MD/Ph.D.

UNIVERSITY:
Type: Public

APPLICATIONS:
Accept Non-Canadians: Yes
Transfers: No
Deferred Admissions: Yes

Primary Application:
OMSAS

Secondary Application: Yes

Early Decision: No

CURRICULUM:
Length: 4-years
Language: English

Dr. Catharine Whiteside - Dean, Faculty of Medicine

CAMPUS:
Office of Admissions &
Student Financial Services
Faculty of Medicine
University of Toronto
Medical Sciences Building,
1 King's College Circle,
Toronto ON M5S 1A8

CONTACT INFORMATION:
Telephone: 416-978-7928
Fax: 416-971-2163

E-Mail: medicine.admiss@utoronto.ca
Website: http://www.md.utoronto.ca

GENERAL INFORMATION:

The University of Toronto was founded in 1843 and is a key part of the second largest healthcare network in North America. The University has two campuses. The St. George campus located in downtown Toronto instructs 205 students while the Mississauga campus instructs 54 students yearly. Students will be informed of their campus allocation upon acceptance. Campus assignments will be for the entire 4-year program and students are able to indicate their preference. A six-year combined MD/PhD program is available.

The mission of the school is preparing future health leaders to contribute to their communities, and to improve the health of individuals and population through the application, discovery, and communications of knowledge.

The curriculum is designed with small-group learning, problem-based learning, lectures, seminars, and laboratory exercises. E-learning is currently being integrated into the curriculum as well. The curriculum is built around seven objectives which are: Medical Expert/Skilled Clinician; Communicator/Doctor-Patient Relationship; Collaborator; Manager; Health Advocate; Scholar; and Professional.

Campus Housing is available.

PREREQUISITES:

A minimum of three years of full-time study is required for admission.

AP/IB: May claim some credit for prerequisite requirements.

Required Courses (laboratory work with science classes is expected):

Life Sciences – 2 years   Humanities – 1 year   Social Sciences 1 - year
Second Language – 1 year

Coursework should provide applicants with an overall understanding of biology, chemistry, physics, and statistics. Statistics is not required, but recommended. Two full courses that have required expository writing are recommended. Applicants are expected to have taken courses at a level that corresponds with their program of study.

<u>MCAT®</u>

MCAT Required: Yes

Average MCAT: 33

Average MCAT Bio: 11.0
Average MCAT Phys: 11.1
Average MCAT Verbal: 10.8
Average MCAT Essay: NA

MCAT minimum: 9/9/9

<u>GPA:</u>

3.94: GPA (overall)
3.6: GPA (minimum)

<u>Combined Programs:</u>

MD/Ph.D.

Testing of Language Proficiency: No, although students must be proficient in English.
MCAT® required: Yes
AMRCB® transcripts are mailed directly to OMSAS for inclusion in the application

CURRICULUM:

Basic Sciences:
The Basic Sciences are taught over 82 weeks using integrated and multidisciplinary content, student-motivated learning, and structured problem-based learning. Patient-Centered learning is the key to the curriculum with small groups tutorials and self-directed work.

Basic Sciences

Year 1	Year 2
The Art and Science of Clinical Medicine 1	The Art and Science of Clinical Medicine 2
Brain and Behavior	Determinants of Community Health
Metabolism and Nutrition	Mechanisms, Manifestations, and Management of Disease
Structure and Function	Family Medicine Longitudinal Experience
Community, Population, and Public Health 1	

Clinical Sciences:
Clinical training takes place at the Baycrest Centre for Geriatric Care, Centre for Addiction and Mental Health, The Hospital for Sick Children, Mount Sinai Hospital, St. Michael's Elizabeth Hospital, Toronto Hospital, Toronto Rehabilitation Institute, Sunnybrook, and Woman's College Health Science Centre.

Clinical Skills

Required Clerkships	Electives and Selectives
Medicine – 6 weeks	Electives – 18 weeks
Surgery – 6 weeks	
Psychiatry – 6 weeks	
Pediatrics – 6 weeks	
OB/GYN – 6 weeks	
Family Medicine – 6 weeks	
Community Medicine – 6 weeks	
Specialty Medicine – 6 weeks	
Specialty Surgery – 6 weeks	
Emergency Medicine – 6 weeks	
Anesthesia – 6 weeks	
Ambulatory and Community Medicine – 6 weeks	

Thesis/Research Required: Optional
Community Service Requirements: Required - through a longitudinal course

TUITION: All currency listings are in Canadian Dollars (CAD)

Canadian Residents: $21,130   International/Visa Students: $62,920
Compulsory Fees: $2,001 (Domestic) / $2,685 (VISA)

Application Fee: OMSAS $210 , secondary application $110
Acceptance Deposit: $1,000 (non-refundable) – applied toward tuition

INTERVIEW:

Interviews: Conducted on weekends in the winter and spring each year. In 2014, 600 applicants were interviewed. Interviews are granted based on file review.

Acceptance Notification: In the spring each year.

SELECTION FACTORS:

Applicants from Canada, the United States, and the international community are all eligible to apply. No preference is given to specific regions or provinces within Canada. All applicants have a calculation of their GPA and are assigned a weighted GPA based on several variables. The minimum GPA is 3.6 for applicants, although a GPA of 3.8 or higher is considered competitive. All applicants must submit results of the Medical College Admission Test (MCAT®) in order to be considered for admission. The MCAT® must have been taken prior to the application deadline and within the past 5 years. MCAT® results from tests taken in excess of five years prior to the current admissions application deadline (October 1st) will not be considered. Only the most recent MCAT® scores will be considered in the application process. A minimum score of 9 in each category is required, and the writing sample is not used in the selection process. Scores below the minimum will jeopardize the success of the application.

The Admissions Committee evaluates multiple non-academic qualities as well in the selection process. An applicant's personal essay, autobiographical sketch, and letters of recommendation are all considered. Applicants are evaluated on their maturity, perseverance, reliability, creativity, leadership, and responsibility. Students must be skilled in collaboration, teamwork, and time management. No specific undergraduate course of study is required, although students are expected to have undergone a rigorous and coherent course of study.

Aboriginal applicants are given additional consideration in the application process, but they must meet the same MCAT®, GPA, and prerequisite requirements as do standard applicants. Applicants who hold a graduate degree have a different set of admission requirements, and a minimum GPA of 3.0 is required for consideration.

Applicant statistics are not reported currently for medical schools located in Ontario.

Western University, Schulich School of Medicine and Dentistry

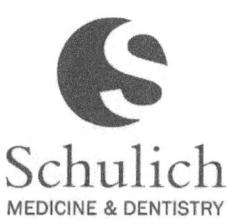

Schulich
MEDICINE & DENTISTRY

Dr. Michael J. Strong - Dean, Schulich School of Medicine and Dentistry

QUICK FACTS

POSITIONS:
171: Total
161: General
3: Aboriginal
3: MD/Ph.D.
3: MD/BSc
1: Oral Maxillofacial surgery program

Average age of 1st year: 23
Male/Female %: 55/45

UNIVERSITY:
Type: Public

APPLICATIONS:
Accept Non-Canadians: No
Transfers: Yes
Deferred Admissions: Yes

Primary Application:
OMSAS

Secondary Application: Yes

Early Decision: No

CURRICULUM:
Length: 4-years
Language: English

CAMPUS:
Admissions
Schulich School of Medicine & Dentistry
Western University
Health Sciences Addition H103
1151 Richmond St.,
London, ON, N6A 5C1

CONTACT INFORMATION:
Telephone: 519-661-3744
Fax: 519-850-2360

E-Mail: admissions.medicine@schulich.uwo.ca
Website: http://www.schulich.uwo.ca/medicine/undergraduate/

GENERAL INFORMATION:

Western University, Schulich School of Medicine and Dentistry was founded in 1881. Western University has two campuses. The main campus is located in London, Ontario and houses 133 students each year. The second campus is located in Windsor, Ontario and houses 38 students each year. Students are able to select their campus of choice and efforts are made to assign students to their campus preference. The education at both campuses is identical. Several combined degrees are available to qualified students.

The mission of the school is to provide outstanding education within a research-intensive environment where tomorrow's physicians, dentists, and health researchers learn to be socially responsible leaders in the advancement of human health.

The curriculum includes small-group learning, supervised clinical experiences, and a blend of lectures and laboratory experiences. The curriculum is designed around a patient-centered focus. The school does have a summer, preparatory program for interested students.

Campus Housing is available.

PREREQUISITES:

Students must have completed a minimum of three years of full-time study prior to applying and are expected to complete a 4-year undergraduate degree prior to matriculation.

Although no specific prerequisite science courses are required, the following are generally expected:

Organic Chemistry – 1 year   Biology – 1 year   Additional Full Science Course – 1 year
Non-Science Courses – 2 full courses of different disciplines and one senior-level course

Testing of Language Proficiency: No, but proficiency in written and spoken English is required.

MCAT®

MCAT Required: Yes

Average MCAT: 29

Average MCAT Bio: 10.0
Average MCAT Phys: 9.0
Average MCAT Verbal: 10.0
Average MCAT Essay: Q

MCAT minimum: 32 combined.

Different individual MCAT requirements are in place for applicants from South-western Ontario

GPA:

3.7: GPA (overall)

Combined Programs:

MD/BSc,
MD/PhD (Western University only)
MD/MSc (Oral Maxillofacial Surgery)

MCAT® required: Yes
AMRCB® transcripts are mailed directly to OMSAS for inclusion in the application

CURRICULUM:

Basic Sciences:

The first two years are dived into six blocks each with a focus on patient-centered education. Facilitators work with students to ensure that students are appropriately progressing through the curriculum. Small group learning, case-based learning, lectures, and laboratory experiences are all utilized.

Basic Sciences

Year 1	Year 2
Introduction to Medicine	Digestive System and Nutrition
Blood	Endocrine and Metabolism
Infection and Immunity	Reproduction
Skin	Key Topics in Family Medicine
Heart and Circulation	Musculoskeletal System
Respiration and Airways	Emergency Care
Genitourinary System	Neurosciences, Eye, and Ear
Physician as Leader	Psychiatry and the Behavioral Sciences
Population Health	Patient Centered Clinical Methods
Epidemiology	Health Care Systems
Medical Ethics and Humanities	Medical Ethics and Humanities
Patient Centered Clinical Methods	Professional Portfolio
Professional Portfolio	

Clinical Sciences:

Students rotate through rural areas of Southwestern Ontario. Electives are available internationally as well if desired.

Clinical Skills

Required Clerkships	Electives and Selectives
Internal Medicine – 12 weeks Surgery – 12 weeks Psychiatry – 6 weeks Pediatrics – 6 weeks OB/GYN – 6 weeks Family Medicine – 6 weeks	Electives – 16 weeks

Thesis/Research Required: Optional
Community Service Requirements: Yes

TUITION: All currency listings are in Canadian Dollars (CAD)

Canadian Residents: $22,929
Compulsory Fees: $973

Application Fee: $100, secondary application fee of $100
Acceptance Deposit: $1,000 (non-refundable) – applied toward tuition

INTERVIEW:

Interviews: Take place in March each year. A total of 473 applicants were interviewed in 2014. The interviews are a structured, standardized interview with a panel of one physician, one senior medical student, and one community representative.

Acceptance Notification: Mailed in May each year.

SELECTION FACTORS:

The Admissions Committee considers Science and Non-Science GPA's, letters of recommendation, essays, extracurricular activities, the exposure to the medical profession, and the MCAT® scores. The MCAT® is required and the test must have been taken within the last 5 years. MCAT® cut-off scores vary each academic year. Only the last set of MCAT® scores are considered for students who have taken the MCAT® more than once. Only students who have achieved the minimum MCAT® scores and GPA will be considered for admission. The personal interview is important in the selection process. Only applicants who are identified as competitive will be invited for an interview.

For applicants from outside of Southwestern Ontario, a minimum GPA of 3.7 is required as are minimum MCAT® scores of: Biological sciences – 12, Physical sciences – 9, Verbal Reasoning – 11. Applicants from Southwestern Ontario must have a minimum GPA of 3.7, and minimum MCAT® scores of: Biological Sciences – 8, Physical Sciences – 8, and Verbal Reasoning – 8, although the combined scores must be at least 32.

The Admissions Committee does not favor any undergraduate program or course of study over others. Community service and extra-curricular activities are important as well. Special consideration is given to residents from specific communities located in Southwestern Ontario. Students from indigenous communities are also given special consideration.

Applicant statistics are not reported currently for medical schools located in Ontario.

Quebec

Université Laval, Faculté de médecine

McGill University, Faculty of Medicine

Université de Montréal, Faculté de médecine

Université de Sherbrooke, Faculté de médecine

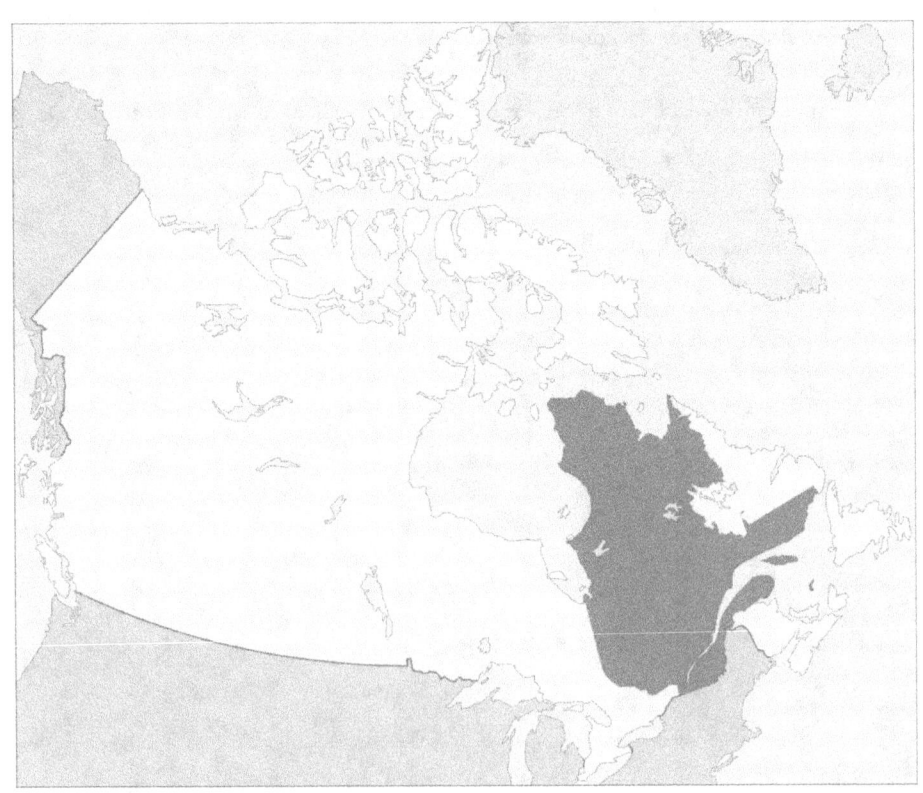

Université Laval, Faculté de médecine

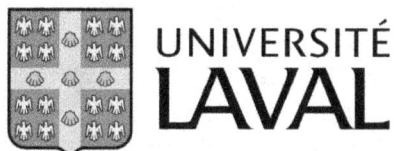

QUICK FACTS

POSITIONS:
227: Total
8:   MD/PhD
6:   Canadian Forces
4:   Aboriginal

UNIVERSITY:
Type: Public

APPLICATIONS:
Accept Non-Canadians: Yes
Transfers: No
Deferred Admissions: No

Application:
Electronic - School Specific

Secondary Application: No

Early Decision: No

CURRICULUM:
Length: 4 year or 5 years
Language: French

Dr. Rénald Bergeron - Doyen, Faculté de médecine

CAMPUS:
Bureau de l'admission
Faculté de médecine
Université Laval,
Pavillon Ferdinand-Vandry Local 2222
Québec QC G1V 0A6

CONTACT INFORMATION:
Telephone: 418-656-2131, ext. 2492
Fax: 418-656-2733

E-Mail: admission@fmed.ulaval.ca
Website: http://www.fmed.ulaval.ca

GENERAL INFORMATION:

Laval University was founded in 1852 and is one of the oldest academic institutions in North America. The medical school is dedicated to the development of high academic standards and research and derives its identify from a mixture of the clinical tradition of French Medicine and the latest advances in North American scientific medicine. Two regional campuses located in Rimouski, Quebec, and Loliette, Quebec are used for regional clerkship locations. The school offers multiple baccalaureate, master's level, and doctoral programs.

The mission of the university is to assure a theoretical and clinical formation which prepares students for practicing medicine competently in a contemporary health system with emphasis on an approach which is scientific, ethical, global, and humanistic.

The curriculum aims to prepare students for a career in any field of medicine. The curriculum uses system-based, large group, and longitudinal courses in the educational process. Educational objectives are structured on communication, collaboration, clinical expertise, eruditions, and professionalism. Several combined degrees are available and research is important for students at the University of Laval. The University does offer a post-baccalaureate program for interested students.

Campus Housing is available.

PREREQUISITES:

A baccalaureate degree or pre-university diploma equivalent to 13 years of the Quebec school systems is required. This may be satisfied by 12 years of pre-university study and one year of advance study.

Required Courses (laboratory work with science coursework is expected):

Chemistry – 3 courses   Biology – 2 courses   Physics – 3 courses
Mathematics – 2 coursers

Testing of Language Proficiency: Yes
MCAT® required: Yes

AMRCB® transcripts: Mail directly to the University.

CURRICULUM:

Basic Sciences:
Basic Science instruction utilized lectures and is organized around anatomical systems.

Basic Sciences
Years 1 and 2
Basic Sciences I, II, and III
Respiratory System: Foundations and clinical problems
Cardiovascular System: Foundations and clinical problems
Physician, Medicine, and Society I, II, III, and IV
Clinical Approach I and II
Digestive System: Foundations and clinical problems
Urinary System and internal environment
Integration I, II, and III
Endocrine System: Foundations and clinical problems
Nervous System: Foundations and clinical problems
Clinical Epidemiology
Senses: Fundamentals and clinical problems
Musculoskeletal System: Foundations and clinical problems
Reproductive system: Foundations and clinical problems
Critical review of the medical literature
Skin covering: rationale and clinical problems
Elderly and end of life care
Normal child and pediatric problems
Mind: rationale and clinical problems
Hematopoietic system: Foundations and clinical problems
Interprofessional person-centered I, II, and III

Clinical Sciences:
Clinical training occurs at Centre Hospitaler de Universite Laval, Hospital de l-enfant-jesus, Hospital du Saint-Sacrement, Hospital Saint-Francois d'Assise, Hotel-Dieu de Levis, Hotel-Dieu de Quebec, and IUCPQ. Two regional campuses are available for clerkship rotations.

Clinical Skills	
Required Clerkships	**Electives and Selectives**
Medicine – 8 weeks Clinical Medicine – 5 weeks Surgery – 8 weeks Psychiatry – 8 weeks Pediatrics – 8 weeks OB/GYN – 8 weeks Family Medicine – 4 weeks Emergency Medicine – 4 weeks	Electives – 20 weeks

Thesis/Research Required: Optional
Community Service Requirements: Optional,

TUITION: All currency listings are in Canadian Dollars (CAD)

Canadian Residents: $10,412   International/Visa Students: $27,186   Quebec Residents: $3,613
Compulsory Fees: $901

MCAT®
MCAT Required: No
Average MCAT: NA

GPA:
Unknown: GPA (overall)

Combined Programs:
MD/PhD

Application Fee: $77
Interview Fee: $100
Acceptance Deposit: None

INTERVIEW:

Interviews: Multiple Mini Interviews (MMI) take place in April each year with 12 short-interview stations. For 2014, 955 applicants were interviewed. An interview fee of $100 is required.

Acceptance Notification: Mailed in May each year.

SELECTION FACTORS:

Applications from Canadian and international applicants are considered, although preference is given to residents of Quebec. A small number of excellent, French-speaking applicants from outside of Quebec are considered each year. The MCAT® is not required at this time. Each year, 2-3 positons may be available for U.S. and international transfer students who are able to start at the clerkship phase of the curriculum.

The Admissions Committee considers essays, extracurricular activities, Science and Non-Science GPA's, and the academic journey. Candidates are considered based on interpersonal skills, character, and overall academic success. The interview is an important part of the selection process and is designed to evaluate different personality characteristics of candidates

Table 1: Laval University Applicant Match Statistics^*

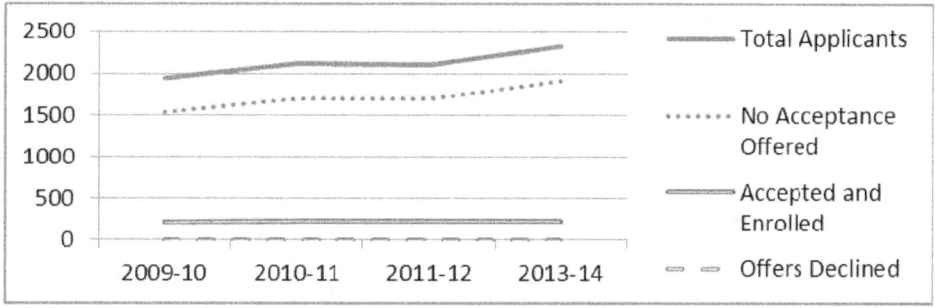

^ Success rate is defined as the percentage of applicants receiving at least one offer of admission regardless of acceptance
* Includes Canadian citizens/landed immigrants who were living outside Canada at time of application
Source: Admission Requirements of Canadian Faculties of Medicine

Table 2: Laval University Applicant Selection Success

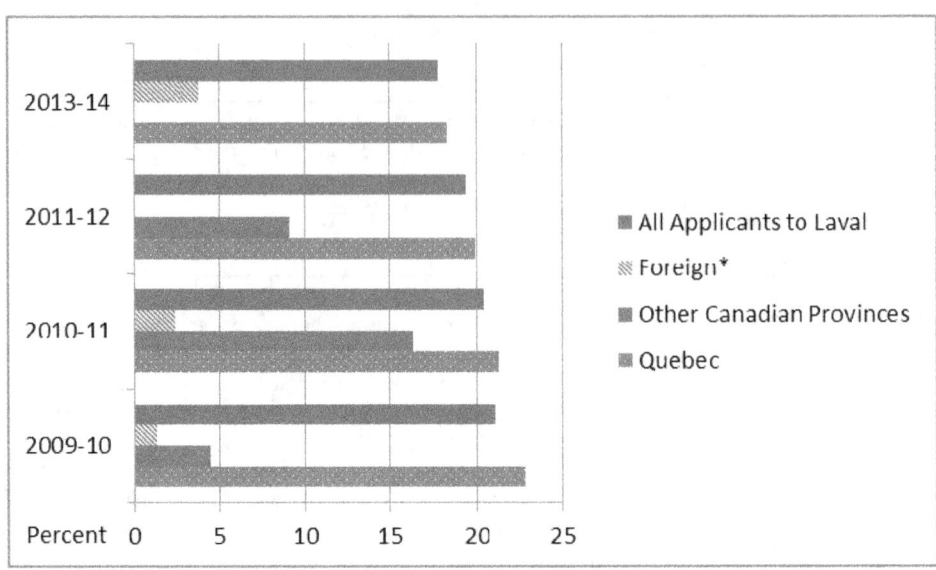

Source: Admission Requirements of Canadian Faculties of Medicine

McGill University, Faculty of Medicine

McGill Faculty of Faculté de
Medicine Médecine

QUICK FACTS

POSITIONS:
184: Total
9: Canadian Residents outside of Quebec
4: Aboriginal Students
4: VISA Students
2: Joint MD/Maxillofacial Surgery Program

75: Preparatory Year

Average age of 1st year: 22
Male/Female %: 45/55

UNIVERSITY:
Type: Public

APPLICATIONS:
Accept Non-Canadians: No
Transfers: No
Deferred Admissions: Yes

Primary Application:
Individual - School Specific

Secondary Application: No

Early Decision: No

CURRICULUM:
Length: 4-years (+1 preparatory)
Language: English

Dr. David Eidelman - Dean, Faculty of Medicine

CAMPUS:
Office of Admissions
Equity and Diversity
Faculty of Medicine
McGill University
1010 Sherbrooke Street West, Suite 1210
Montréal QC H3A 2R7

CONTACT INFORMATION:
Telephone: 514-398-3517
Fax: 514-398-4631

E-Mail: admissions.med@mcgill.ca
Website: http://www.mcgill.ca/medadmissions

GENERAL INFORMATION:

McGill University Faculty of Medicine was originally founded in 1821 and was the first medical school founded in Canada. Students come to McGill from over 150 countries. The University has a preparatory (Med-P) program and the MD-CEM programs. The majority of students in the preparatory program are admitted to the M.D.-C.E.M. program upon completion of one-year of study. Each year, 75 students are admitted to the Preparatory program

The mission of the school is the advancement of learning through scholarship, teaching, and service to society by offering the best education available, carrying out internationally-recognized scholarly activities, and providing service to society. The desire of the school is to provide a solid foundation in the humanistic skills required to be an outstanding physician.

The curriculum is designed to prepare students to meet the highest standard of medical professionalism and practice. Small-group learning, lectures, computer-based teaching, and laboratories are all utilized. Several joint degree programs are available for interested students including MD/MBA and MD/PhD programs.

Campus Housing is available for co-ed residents as well as a woman's residence.

PREREQUISITES:

A Bachelor's degree is required for Admission to the MD Program. Applicants with a Diplôme d'études collégiales, may apply with 90-credits from a Quebec university.

A College d'enseignement general et professional (CEGEP) diploma is required at the time of admission to the preparatory program.

Preparatory Program Prerequisites:

Required Courses (laboratory work with science coursework is expected):
General Chemistry – 1 year   Organic Chemistry – 1/2 year   General Biology – 1 year
General Physics – 1 year

MD Program Prerequisites:
Laboratory work is expected with all science courses.
General Biology – 1 year   General Chemistry – 1 year   General Physics – 1 year
Organic Chemistry – 1 course

MCAT®

MCAT Required: Variable

Average MCAT: 30

Average MCAT Bio: 11.0
Average MCAT Phys: 11.0
Average MCAT Verbal: 10.0
Average MCAT Essay: P

MCAT Minimum: 27 to be considered

GPA:

3.80: GPA (overall)

3.5. Minimum GPA

Combined Programs:
MD-CM/MBA, MD-CM/PhD, MD-CM/OMFS

Courses in physiology, biochemistry, cellular and molecular biology, and statistics are recommended.

Testing of Language Proficiency: No
The MCAT® is required for VISA students and Canadian citizens or permanent residents who have graduated from non-Canadian institutions.
AMRCB® transcripts: Mailed directly to school.

Pass/fail grades are not acceptable and basic science courses completed more than 8 years ago must be repeated. Exception may be made for applicants with advanced degrees in the material concerned.

CURRICULUM:

The overall curriculum is designed with four components which are Basis of Medicine, Introduction to Clinical Medicine, Practice of Medicine, and Back to Basics. The curriculum uses a multi-disciplinary approach for the basic and clinical sciences.

Basic Sciences:

Basic Sciences	
Year 1	**Year 1**
Molecules to Global Health	Reproduction and Sexuality
Respiration	Human Behavior
Circulation	OSCE
Renal	
Digestion and Metabolism	
Defense	
Infection	
Movement	

Clinical Sciences:
Clinical instruction takes place at Douglas Hospital, Montreal Children's Hospital, Montreal General Hospital, Montreal Neurological Hospital, Royal Victoria Hospital, and Sir Mortimer B. Davies-Jewish General Hospital as well as other affiliated teaching sites. A one-year integrated clerkship is available in Gatineau, ON.

Clinical Sciences	
Required Clerkships	**Electives and Selectives**
Medicine – 8 weeks	Selectives – 4 week Public Health
Surgery – 8 weeks	
Psychiatry – 8 weeks	Electives – 12 weeks
Pediatrics – 8 weeks	
OB/GYN – 8 weeks	
Family Medicine – 8 weeks	
Geriatric Medicine – 4 weeks	
Emergency Medicine – 4 weeks	

Thesis/Research Required: Optional
Community Service Requirements: Optional

TUITION: All currency listings are in Canadian Dollars (CAD)

Preparatory Year

Canadian Residents: $2,273   Quebec Residents: $2,273   International/VISA Residents: $38,531
Compulsory Fees: $1,689

MD Program

Canadian Residents: $13,946   International/Visa Students: $35,988   Quebec Residents: $4,774
Compulsory Fees: $2,080

Application Fee: $140

International students are subject to additional health insurance fees.
Acceptance Deposit: $500 (non-refundable) – applied toward tuition

INTERVIEW:

Interviews: Multiple Mini Interviews (MMI) take place in April each year.   In 2014, 190 applicants were interviewed for the MD program. Interviews can be held in either French or English.

Acceptance Notification: E-mailed and posted electronically mid-May each year.

SELECTION FACTORS:

Applications are considered for Canadian citizens and from the U.S. and international community. International (non-U.S.) Medical Graduates may apply for advanced standing. The MCAT® is required for all applicants from out-of-province, for international applicants, and where the basis of admission is from a non-Canadian university.   The MCAT® is optional for out-of-province and from international graduates whose degree is from a Canadian University. The MCAT® is not required for International Medical Graduates who have completed the Medical Council of Canada's Equivalence Exam, non-traditional applicants, or for application to the Med-P program. The highest overall score on the MCAT® is considered if the test has been taken more than once. An MCAT® score of 30 or higher is considered competitive.

Students are given a weighted GPA based on several variables. Variability exists with the GPA weighting system depending on the background and geographic location of the applicant. Accepted students generally have a GPA of 3.8 or higher. A GPA of 3.5 or higher is required in order to be considered for admission.

The Admission Committee considers extracurricular activities, personal characteristics, essays, and exposure to the medical profession. Students are sought who are compassionate, insightful, honest, creative, curious, and who display a respect for others. Students are expected to be reliable, dependable, and be able to accept responsibility and leadership. Letters of recommendation and the personal interview are important in the selection process. Science and Non-Science GPA's are both considered and the MCAT® scores are important. Applicants should have strong academic qualifications and achievements. No specific field of study is favored over any other. Applicants are selected based on their academic success and the personal interview. Special consideration may be given to First Nation/Inuit applicants who are residents of Quebec.

Table 1: McGill University Applicant Match Statistics – Preparatory Program^*

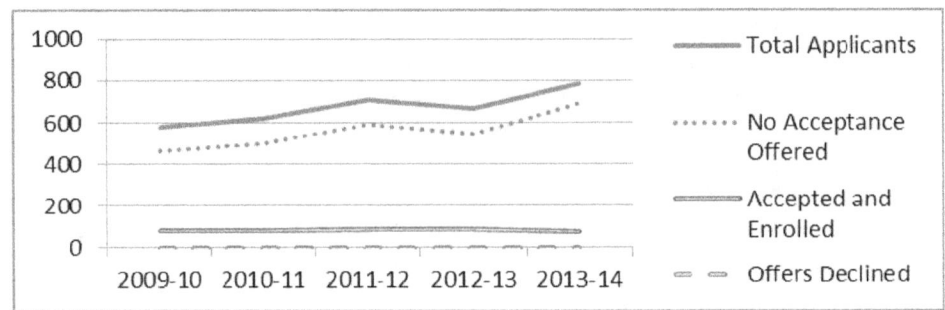

^ Success rate is defined as the percentage of applicants receiving at least one offer of admission regardless of acceptance
* Includes Canadian citizens/landed immigrants who were living outside Canada at time of application
Source: Admission Requirements of Canadian Faculties of Medicine

Table 2: McGill University Applicant Selection Success - Preparatory Year

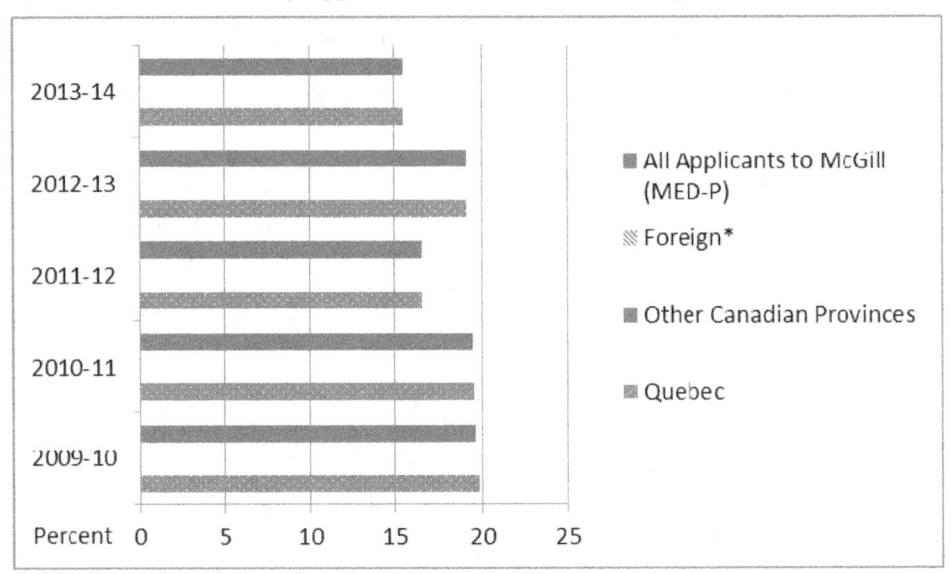

Source: Admission Requirements of Canadian Faculties of Medicine

Table 1: McGill University Applicant Match Statistics- MD-CM Program^*

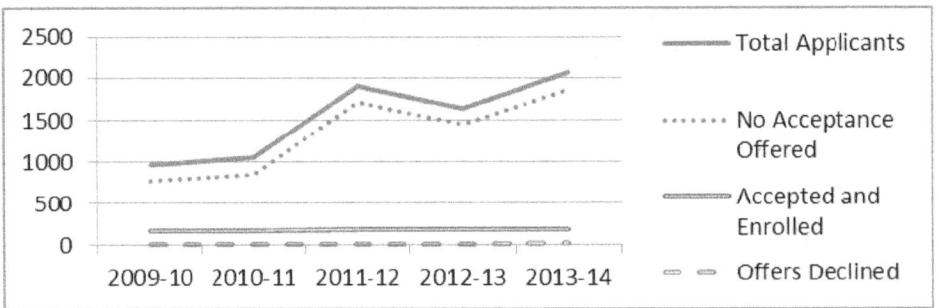

^ Success rate is defined as the percentage of applicants receiving at least one offer of admission regardless of acceptance
* Includes Canadian citizens/landed immigrants who were living outside Canada at time of application
Source: Admission Requirements of Canadian Faculties of Medicine

Table 2: McGill University Applicant Selection Success - MD-CM Program

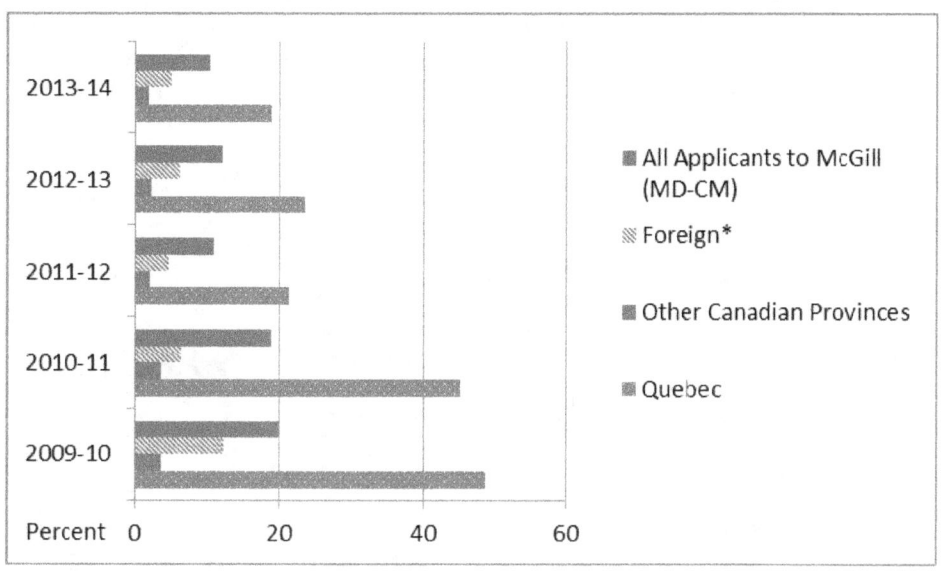

Source: Admission Requirements of Canadian Faculties of Medicine

Université de Montréal, Faculté de médecine

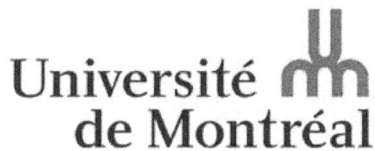

Université de Montréal

Dr. Hélène Boisjoly - Doyenne, Faculté de médecine

CAMPUS:
Université de Montréal
CP 6205, succursale Centre-ville,
Faculty of Medicine & Dentistry
Montréal QC H3C 3T5

CONTACT INFORMATION:
Telephone: 514-343-7076
Fax: 514-343-5788

E-Mail: admissions-info@sar.umontreal.ca 1-002 Katz
Website: http://www.umontreal.ca

QUICK FACTS

POSITIONS:
295: Total
285: Quebec Residents
213: Med-P
6: Canadian Forces
4: Aboriginal

Male/Female %: 40/60

UNIVERSITY:
Type: Public

APPLICATIONS:
Accept Non-Canadians: Yes
Transfers: No
Deferred Admissions: No

Primary Application:
Individual – school specific

Secondary Application: No

Early Decision: No

CURRICULUM:
Length: 4-years
Language: French

GENERAL INFORMATION:

The Faculty of Medicine of the Universite de Montreal was first established in 1878 and is the second largest university in Canada. The medical school was formally a branch of the University of Laval. The main campus is located in Montreal which houses approximately 240 students. A satellite campus is located in Trois-Rivieres which houses approximately 40 students each year, most of which are in the premedical phase, although a student can complete the entire medical curriculum in this location if desired.

The mission of the University is to provide medical knowledge, clinical skills, and professional attitudes through its undergraduate medical program so that students will be able to enter postgraduate training in any field of medicine including teaching, research, and health care management. The school prepares students to be leaders, communicators, collaborators, and promoters of health.

A 5-year combined preparatory program is offers as well, and 4-year and 5-year students are assigned to both campus locations. Several combined degree programs are available as well. International applicants and those without appropriate prerequisite courses must enroll in the preparatory year 5-year program. The curriculum utilizes problem-based learning and system-based, interdisciplinary learning.

Campus Housing is available.

PREREQUISITES:

A minimum of two years of college from a Collège d'enseignement general et professionnel (CÉGEP) is required to apply. Alternately, a college degree with completion of the required prerequisites prior to admission is required.

Required Courses (laboratory work with science coursework is expected):

Chemistry – 3 courses   Organic Chemistry – 1 year   Biology – 2 courses
Physics – 3 courses   English – 1 year   Mathematics (through Trigonometry) – 2 courses

Additional prerequisites include philosophy, behavioral science, social sciences, and French.

Testing of Language Proficiency:
MCAT® required: No

<u>MCAT®</u>

MCAT Required: No

<u>GPA:</u>

GPA : Not published:

<u>Combined Programs:</u>

Public Health, Health Administration, other

AMRCB® transcripts: Mailed directly to school.

CURRICULUM:

Basic Sciences:
Instruction uses a competency-based approach and teaches inter-professional collaborative practices. Simulation labs are used throughout the program as are small groups and problem-based learning.

Basic Sciences

Year 1	Year 2
Microbiology and Virology	Introduction to Clinical Medicine
Introduction to clinical anatomy	Growth, Development and Aging
General Physiology	Pathology and Immunology
Cell and Tissue Biology	Microbiology and Infectious Disease
Awareness of the Patient and Family, part 1	Hematology
Molecular Biology of the Cell	Neurology
Basic Notions in Ethics	Clinical Epidemiology
Nutrition and Metabolism	Heart and Circulation
Medical Pharmacology	Breathing and Oxygenation
Quantitative Methods in Medicine	Kidney and Urinary Tract
Awareness of the Patient and Family, part 2	Digestion and Nutrition
Medical Genetics	Endocrinology and Metabolism
Human Embryology	Multisystem Problems
Development of the Psychic System	Psychic Sciences
Social Aspects of Health	Musculoskeletal

Clinical Sciences:
Clinical training takes place at Centre Hospitalier Cote-des-Niegres, Centre Hospitalier de Verdun, Cite de la sante de Laval, Institute de Cardiologie de Montreal, Institute de Rancherches Clinique de Montreal, Institute Philppe-Pinelde Montreal, Institute de Readaptation de Montreal, Hospital Louis-H Lafontaine, Hospital Maisonneuvre-Rosemont, Hospital Notre-Dame, Hospital Riviere-des-Praries, Hospital du Sacre-Couer de Montreal, Hospital Saint-Justine, Hospital Saint-Luc, and Hotel-Dieu de Montréal,

Clinical Skills

Required Clerkships	Electives and Selectives
Medicine – 8 weeks	Electives – 8 weeks
Surgery – 8 weeks	
Psychiatry – 8 weeks	Selectives
Pediatrics – 8 weeks	Medical or Pediatrics – 8 weeks
OB/GYN – 8 weeks	Surgical Subspecialties – 8 weeks
Family Medicine – 4 weeks	
Radiology – 4 weeks	
Geriatrics – 4 weeks	
Community Medicine – 4 weeks	
Anesthesiology – 2 weeks	
Ophthalmology – 2 weeks	

Thesis/Research Required: Optional
Community Service Requirements: Optional

TUITION: All currency listings are in Canadian Dollars (CAD)

Canadian Residents: $9,145   International/VISA Residents: $24,482   Quebec Residents: $3,262
Compulsory Fees: $1,220

Application Fee: $115
Acceptance Deposit: $200 (non-refundable) – applied toward tuition

INTERVIEW:

Interviews: Multiple Mini Interviews (MMI) take place in April each year.   Regional interviews are available for Maritimes residents only.   An interview fee of $100 is in place. Approximately one-third of applicants are interviewed each year.

Acceptance Notification: Mailed mid-May each year.

SELECTION FACTORS:

Applicants are accepted from Canadian Citizens, landed immigrants, and highly qualified French-Speaking applicants from the United States and international community.   The Admissions Committee seeks competitive candidates and a global score for each applicant is derived from the academic record and interviews.   The overall academic performance of applicants is important as is the personal interview in the selection process.   For applicants with a PhD, research performance can be an important factor for selection as well.   Preference is given to applicants from Quebec.

All applicants have a performance rating calculated that is used in the selection process.   The MCAT® is not required.   Applicants are expected to have a competitive GPA.

All applicants apply to the preparatory year for the MD program.   The Admissions Committee decides if an applicant is placed in the preparatory program or directly into the MD program based on their academic profile.   Approximately 75% of the applicants are placed in the preparatory program.   Approximately one-third of all applicants are invited for an interview.

Table 1: Montreal University Applicant Match Statistics – Preparatory Program^*

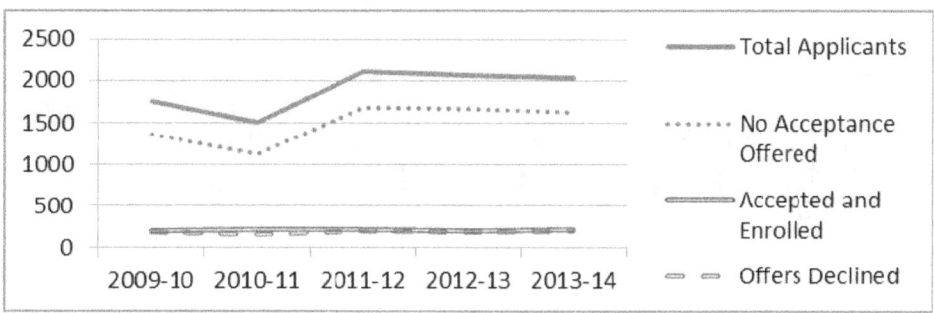

^ Success rate is defined as the percentage of applicants receiving at least one offer of admission regardless of acceptance
* Includes Canadian citizens/landed immigrants who were living outside Canada at time of application
Source: Admission Requirements of Canadian Faculties of Medicine

Table 2: Montreal University Applicant Match Statistics – MD Program^*

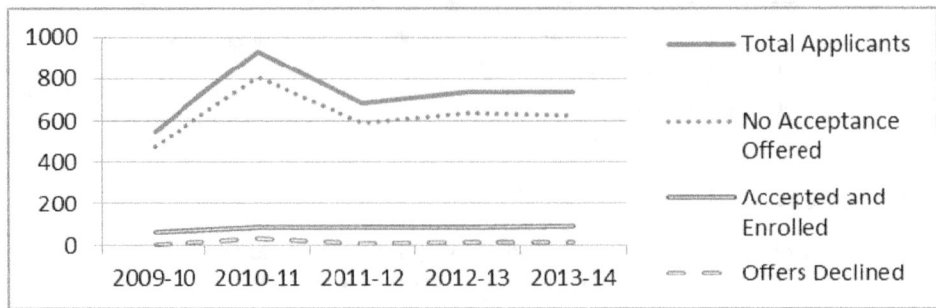

^ Success rate is defined as the percentage of applicants receiving at least one offer of admission regardless of acceptance
* Includes Canadian citizens/landed immigrants who were living outside Canada at time of application
Source: Admission Requirements of Canadian Faculties of Medicine

Table 3: Montreal University Applicant Selection Success - Preparatory Program

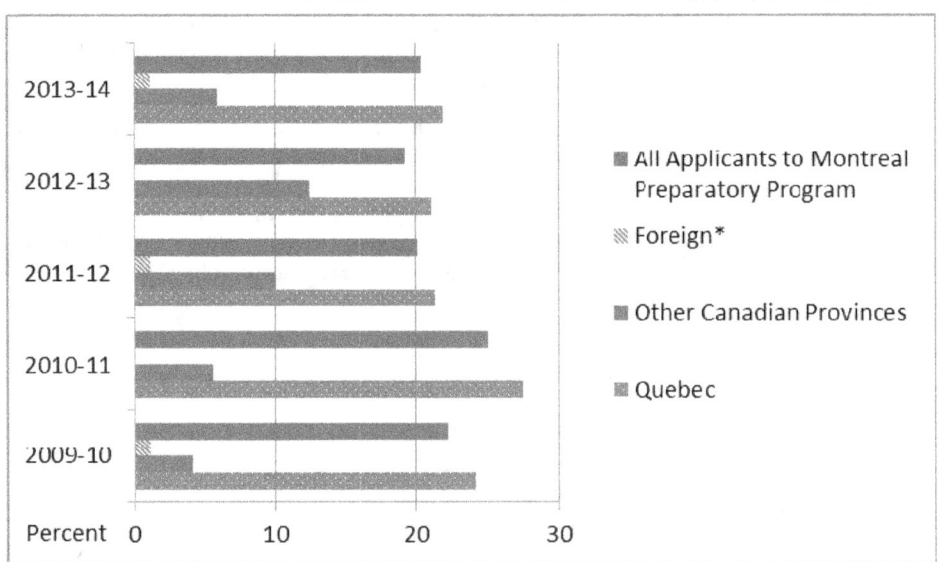

Source: Admission Requirements of Canadian Faculties of Medicine

Table 4: Montreal University Applicant Selection Success - MD Program

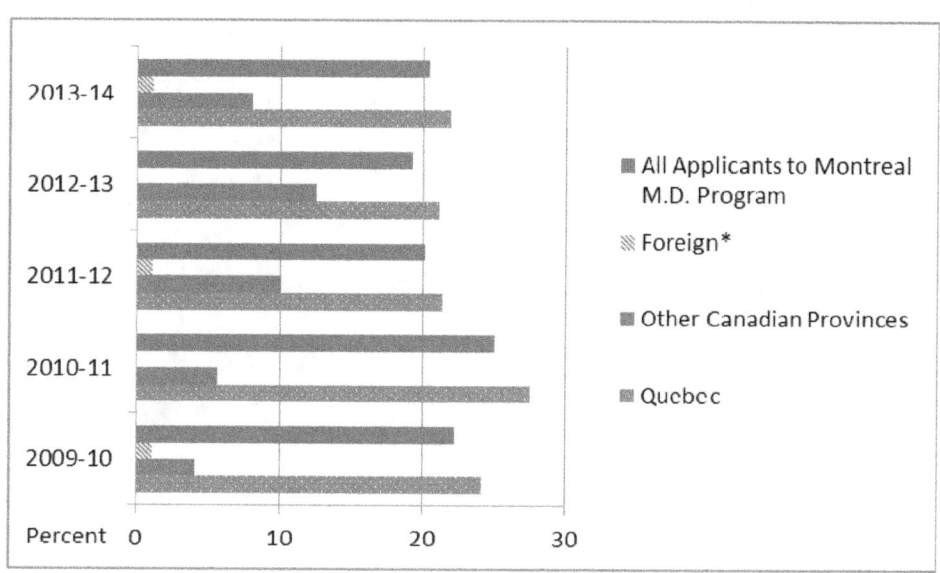

Source: Admission Requirements of Canadian Faculties of Medicine

Université de Sherbrooke, Faculté de médecine

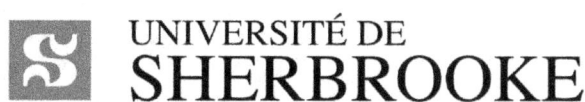

Dr. Pierre Cossette - Doyen, Faculté de médecine et des sciences de la santé

CAMPUS:
Bureau de la registraire
Université de Sherbrooke
2500, boulevard de Université,
Sherbrooke QC J1K 2R1

CONTACT INFORMATION:
Telephone: 819-821-7688
Fax: 819-821-7966

E-Mail: infoadm@usherbrooke.ca
Website: http://www.usherbrooke.ca/doctorat_medecine

QUICK FACTS

POSITIONS:
207: Total
169: Quebec Residents
30: Atlantic Canada Residents
2: Western Canada Residents
2: Foreign Students
1: Aboriginal

Male/Female %: 40/60

UNIVERSITY:
Type: Public

APPLICATIONS:
Accept Non-Canadians: No
Transfers: No
Deferred Admissions: No

Application: School Specific - Electronic or Paper

Secondary Application: Yes

Early Decision: No

CURRICULUM:
Length: 4-years
Language: French

GENERAL INFORMATION:

The University of Sherbrooke Faculty of Medicine was founded in 1966 and over 40,000 students are enrolled in the University in all fields of study. The medical school currently operates three campuses located in Sherbrooke, Saguenay, and Moncton. The Sherbrooke campus hosts 173 students, Sagueny hosts 33 students, and Moncton hosts 26 students. The Moncton site is only for New Brunswick applicants.

The mission of the school is to improve the health and well-being of people and populations through education, clinical services, knowledge transfer, and education. The curriculum utilizes small-groups and problem-based learning and the education process is integrated through the curriculum. Several combined degrees are available for motivated students.

Campus housing is available.

PREREQUISITES:

The minimum requirement for admission is 75 university credits prior to the application being filed or a 2-year degree. It is expected that a diploma or degree equivalent to the college student diploma (CEGEP) given by the Quebec Ministry of Education will have been obtained prior to the start of studies.

General Chemistry – 3 courses   General Biology – 2 courses   Physics – 3 courses
Mathematics (through Calculus) – 2 courses   Organic Chemistry – 1 year

Applicants are expected to have coursework in in the Humanities and the Social Sciences as well.

Testing of Language Proficiency: No, but applicants must be fluent in French.
MCAT® required: No   .
AMRCB® transcripts: Mailed directly to school.

CURRICULUM:

Basic Sciences:
The educational process involves case studies, small-group discussions, hand-on experience, and computer-based learning. The program is divided into three phases.

MCAT®

MCAT Required: No

GPA:

Unknown: GPA (overall)

Combined Programs:

MD/MSc, MD/PhD

Basic Sciences

Phase I	Phase II	Phase III
Biomedical Sciences Units I and II	Integration of Basic and Clinical Sciences	Reasoning and Clinical Skills
	System Based Educational Blocks	Multidisciplinary Units Internal Medicine Pediatrics Surgery Psychiatry Obstetrics and Gynecology

Clinical Sciences:

Clinical rotations occur at several hospitals including Cuse Bowen, Cuse Fleurimont, George L. Dumont Hospital. Hospital Charles Le Mayne, and Hospital Saint-Croix. Students must spend at least one-third of their clinical clerkships in a rural location.

Clinical Skills – Phase IV

Required Clerkships	Electives and Selectives
Medicine – 10.5 weeks Surgery – 7 weeks Psychiatry – 7 weeks Pediatrics – 7 weeks OB/GYN – 7 weeks Family Medicine – 7 weeks Emergency Medicine – 7 weeks Community Health – 4 weeks Multidisciplinary* – 3.5 weeks	Selectives – 8 weeks Specialized Medicine Specialized Surgery Specialized Pediatrics Electives – 12 weeks

*Multidisciplinary include a combination of Anesthesia, Dermatology,
and Ophthalmology,

Thesis/Research Required: No
Community Service Requirements: Optional

TUITION: All currency listings are in Canadian Dollars (CAD)

Canadian Residents: $10,824   International/Visa Students: $28,003   Quebec Residents: $4,287
Compulsory Fees: $1,030

Application Fee: $70
Acceptance Deposit: $300 (non-refundable) – applied toward tuition

INTERVIEW:

Interviews: Occur in April every year. Multiple Mini Interviews (MMI) and the Test d'aptitude à l'apprentissage de la médecine à Université de Sherbrooke (TAAMUS) are given to all applicants. The TAAMUS is a paper test given over an hour. In 2014, 810 applicants from Quebec and 75 applicants from Atlantic provinces were interviewed. Video interviews are available for international students..

Acceptance Notification: Mailed May through August each year

SELECTION FACTORS:

Selected students are chosen based on academic performance as well as personality traits. An overall academic score is developed for each students based on multiple criteria. The interview is an important part of the selection process. Priority is given to applicants from Quebec and those from rural or remote areas. Fifteen positions are reserved for applicants form New Brunswick and one position is reserved for and applicant from Prince Edward Island, and Nova Scotia. Two positions are reserved for applicants from foreign countries. Applicants must be fluent in spoken and written French.

The MCAT® is not required for admission. If the MCAT® was taken, it is not considered in the admission process. All applicants are expected to have a competitive GPA and have completed a rigorous course of study.

Table 1: Sherbrooke University Applicant Match Statistics^*

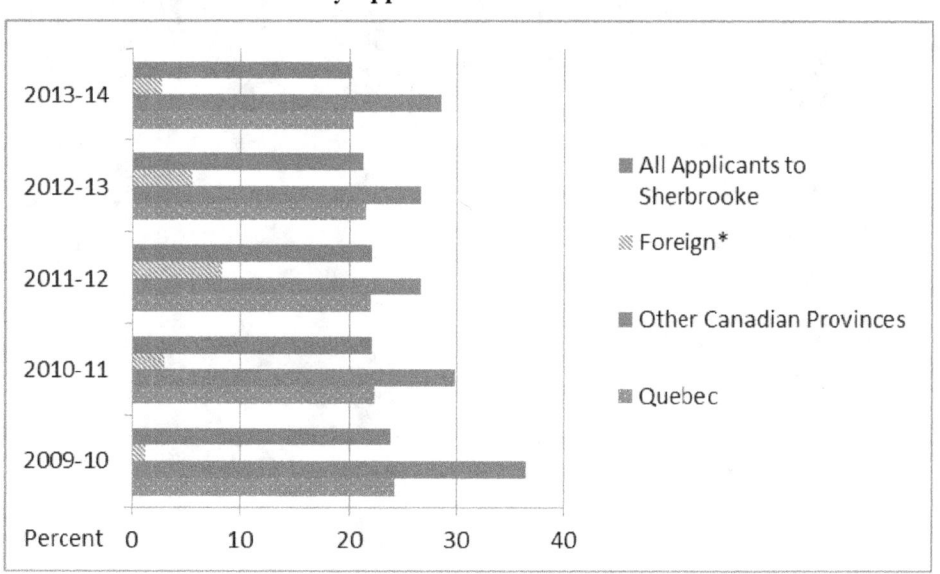

^ Success rate is defined as the percentage of applicants receiving at least one offer of admission regardless of acceptance
* Includes Canadian citizens/landed immigrants who were living outside Canada at time of application
Source: Admission Requirements of Canadian Faculties of Medicine

Table 2: Sherbrooke University Applicant Selection Success

Source: Admission Requirements of Canadian Faculties of Medicine

Saskatchewan

University of Saskatchewan, College of Medicine

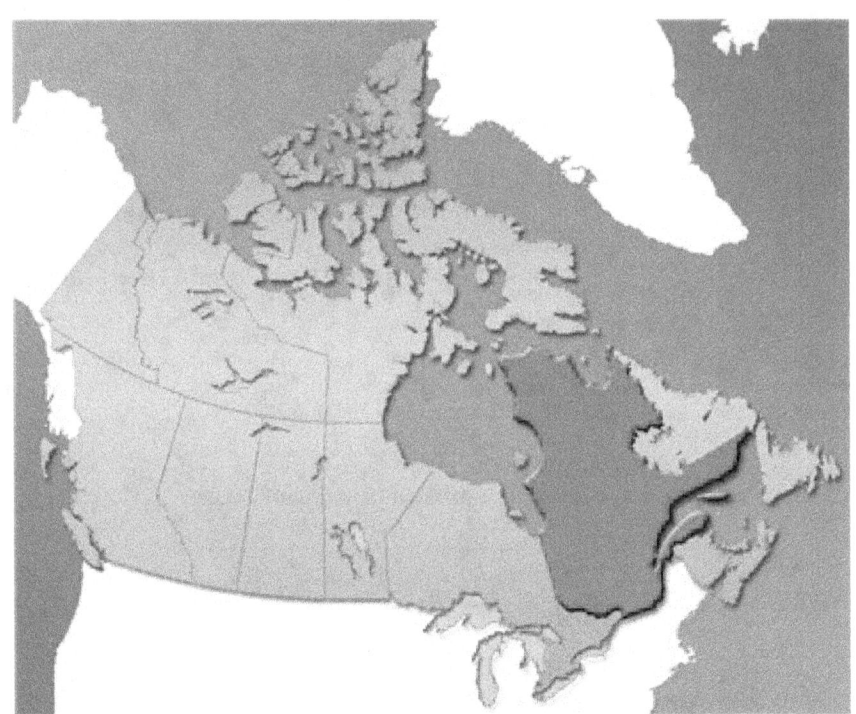

University of Saskatchewan, College of Medicine

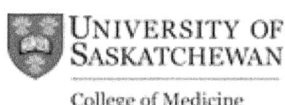

QUICK FACTS

POSITIONS:
100: Total
10: Out-of-province
10: Aboriginal

Average age of 1st year: 23

UNIVERSITY:
Type: Public

APPLICATIONS:
Accept Non-Canadians: No
Transfers: No
Deferred Admissions: Yes

Primary Application:
Individual – School Specific

Secondary Application: No

Early Decision: No

CURRICULUM:
Length: 4-years
Language: English

Dr. Preston Smith - Dean, College of Medicine

CAMPUS:
University of Saskatchewan
College of Medicine
5D40 Health Sciences Building
107 Wiggins Rd.
Saskatoon SK S7N 5E5

CONTACT INFORMATION:
Telephone: 306-966-4030
Fax: 306-966-2601

E-Mail: med.admissions@usask.ca
Website: http://www.medicine.usask.ca/admission

GENERAL INFORMATION:

The University of Saskatchewan was founded in 1926 with the present college structure having started in 1956. The college has a full range of academic programs and has over 20,000 enrolled students. The university strives to enable medical students to develop the skills, knowledge, attitudes, and values that will provide the foundation necessary to become a practicing physician. The curriculum is designed to allow graduates to pursue a career in any field of medicine and utilizes a distributed medical education model.

Two combined programs are available. An MD/PhD program is available but open only to those who have already been accepted to the MD program. An MBA/MD program is available for successful applicants to the MD program who defer admission for one year to complete an MBA program. The objective of the undergraduate medical curriculum is to allow physicians to become medical experts, health advocates, learners, collaborators, a resource managers, and communicators.

Campus Housing is available.

PREREQUISITES:

Saskatchewan Applicants
Students must have completed the required prerequisite coursework, or have taken the MCAT® and have completed a baccalaureate degree prior to admission. If meeting the prerequisite requirements, students must have taken all coursework at the University of Regina or the University of Saskatchewan within the last five years.

Out-of-Province Applicants
Students are required to complete the MCAT® and have a 4-year baccalaureate degree. Students may apply after 90 credits have been completed during the preceding 36 months. Out-of-province students must apply only after or during the last year of their four year degree. The baccalaureate degree must have been started within the last five years prior to the application.

MCAT®

MCAT Required: Yes (unless a Saskatchewan resident who meets the prerequisite requirements)

Average MCAT: 33

Average MCAT Bio: 11.0
Average MCAT Phys: 11.0
Average MCAT Verbal: 10.0
Average MCAT Essay: Q

Minimum MCAT for Saskatchewan Residents: 26 with no section <8

Minimum MCAT for Out-of-Province Applicants: 30, with no section <8

GPA:

89.48%: GPA (overall)

78%: Saskatchewan Resident minimum GPA

83%: Non-Saskatchewan Resident minimum GPA

Combined Programs:
MD/PhD, MBA/MD

Prerequisites include:

Biochemistry – 1 year	Biology – 1year	General Chemistry – 1 year
Organic chemistry – 1 year	Physics – 1 year	English – 1 year
Social Sciences and Humanities 1 year		

Testing of Language Proficiency: No
MCAT® required: Yes
AMRCB® transcripts: Mailed directly to school.

CURRICULUM:

The overall curriculum seeks to integrate the basic and clinical sciences throughout the education process. A problem-solving approach organized by body systems is utilized. The curriculum is divided into four phases.

Basic Sciences:

The Basic Science include instruction with problem-based learning, systems and case-based learning, independent learning, and early patient interaction.

Basic Sciences

Year 1	Year 2	
Phase A	Phase B	Phase C
Basic Biomedical Sciences • Physiology • Embryology • Anatomy • Histology	Microbiology and Pharmacology/Therapeutics	Occupational/Environmental Health
Nutrition, Neurosciences, Genetics and Basic Pathological Concepts	The Determinants of Health for Individuals and Specific Groups	Canada's Healthcare System
Clinical Medicine	Professional Skills Sessions	Clinical Epidemiology and Preventive Medicine
		Professional Skills Sessions

Clinical Sciences:

Clinical Clerkships take place at the General Hospital in Regina, Royal University, in Saskatchewan Health Region, St. Paul's City Hospital, and Saskatoon City Hospital. Students will be assigned a core set of rotations centered either in the Regina/Qu'Appelle Health Region or in the Saskatoon Health Region. Approximately one third of students are based at the Regina site for clerkships.

Clinical Skills

Required Clerkships	Electives and Selectives
Internal Medicine – 12 weeks Surgery – 8 weeks Psychiatry – 6 weeks Pediatrics – 6 weeks OB/GYN – 6 weeks Family Medicine – 6 weeks Emergency Medicine – 2 weeks Anesthesiology – 2 weeks	Electives – 12 weeks

Thesis/Research Required: Optional
Community Service Requirements: Optional

TUITION: All currency listings are in Canadian Dollars (CAD)

Canadian Residents: $15,530
Compulsory Fees: $785.95

Application Fee: $125
Acceptance Deposit: 10% of tuition (non-refundable) – applied toward tuition

INTERVIEW:

Interviews: Multiple Mini Interviews (MMI) take place in March each year. A total of 322 applicants were interviewed in 2014 of which 217 were Saskatchewan residents and 51 were other residents of Canada.

Acceptance Notification: E-mailed in May each year.

SELECTION FACTORS:

Only Canadian citizens, landed immigrants and visa holders are eligible to apply. Preference is given to Saskatchewan residents. The Admissions Committee considers the Science and Non-Science GPA's and the MCAT® score. The essay, extracurricular activities, exposure to the medical profession, and letters of recommendation are also considered. The overall academic qualifications of each applicant are considered as are the individual personal qualities. Grades from graduate degree programs are not considered. The interview is an important part of the selection process.

Saskatchewan residents should have an overall GPA average of 78% or greater and no individual course grade below 60%. The MCAT® is not required for Saskatchewan residents that have completed all the prerequisite requirements. For those who have not completed all the requirements, the MCAT® should be taken and a minimum score of 26 is required with no individual sections with scores of less than 8.

Out-of-province applicants are expected to have a minimum GPA of at least 83%. MCAT® scores must be from one sitting and a score of a 30 or above is required with no section with scores of less than 8. MCAT® must have been taken within the last 5 years.

Aboriginal students may apply through the Aboriginal Equity Access Program. Aboriginal students must still meet the same acceptance requirements as other students, but only compete for positions within the Aboriginal applicant program. Aboriginal applicants may apply under the prerequisite requirements even if coursework was taken outside of Saskatchewan.

Table 1: University of Saskatchewan Applicant Match Statistics^*

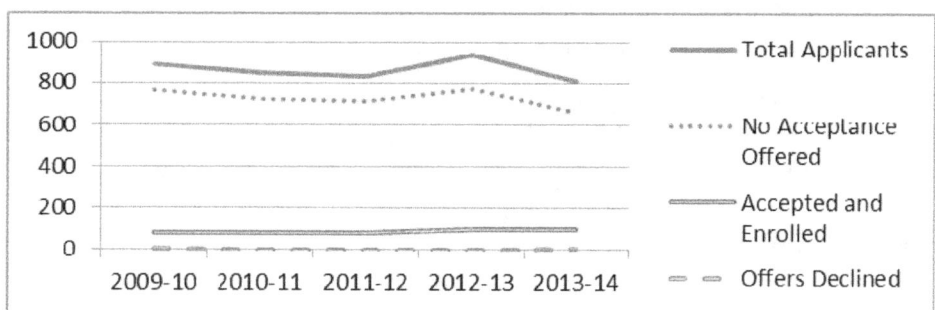

^ Success rate is defined as the percentage of applicants receiving at least one offer of admission regardless of acceptance
* Includes Canadian citizens/landed immigrants who were living outside Canada at time of application
Source: Admission Requirements of Canadian Faculties of Medicine

Table 2: University of Saskatchewan Applicant Selection Success

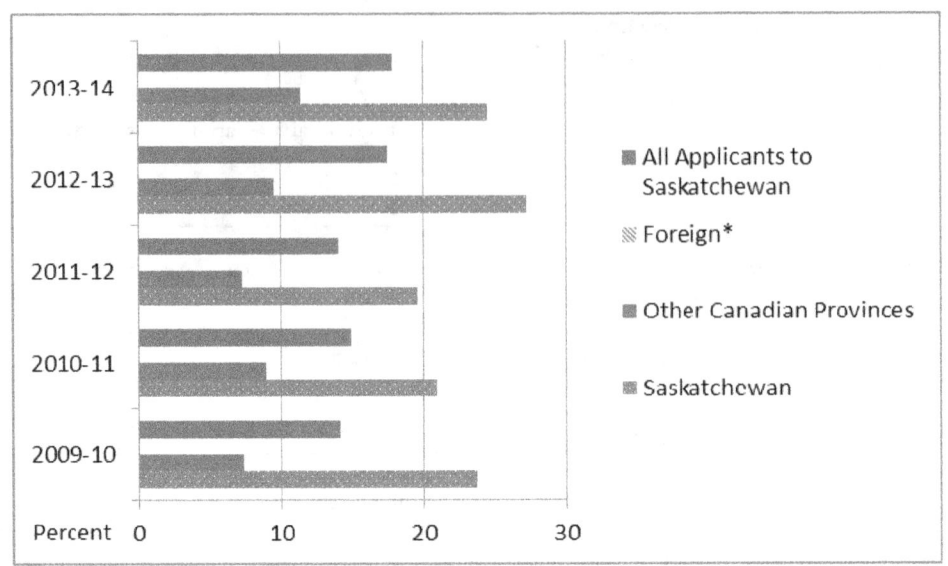

Source: Admission Requirements of Canadian Faculties of Medicine

Former Medical School in Canada

Medical School	Province	City	Est.	Closed	Degree	Notes
Kingston Woman's Medical Card	Ontario	Kingston	1883	1893	MD	Historically affiliated with Queen's University
Laval University Medical Faculty	Quebec	Montreal	1878	1891	MD	Absorbed by Montreal School of Medicine and Surgery in 1891
Ontario Medical College for Women	Ontario	Toronto	1883	1906	MD	Historically affiliated with University of Toronto
St. Lawrence School of Medicine	Quebec	St. Lawrence	1851	1852	MD	
Toronto School of Medicine	Ontario	Toronto	1847	1887	MD	-Historically affiliated with University of Toronto and Victoria University. -Absorbed in 1887 by University of Toronto
Trinity Medical College	Ontario	Toronto	1853	1903	MD	-1853 Upper Canada School of Medicine -1870 reorganized as Faculty of Medicine of Trinity College -1877 became independent Trinity Medical College -1878 affiliated with Trinity University and University of Toronto -1903 merged with the University of Toronto
University of Bishop College Faculty of Medicine	Quebec	Montreal	1870	1905	MD	-Absorbed by McGill University in 1905
Victoria University Medical Department	Ontario	Toronto	1853	1869	MD	-Absorbed by University of Toronto in 1902 -Also known as Rolph's School in past

Source: Council on Medical Education and Hospitals. American Medical Association, 1918

REFERENCES

Admissions Requirements of Canadian Faculties of Medicine - Admission in 2015

Alberta IMG Association

American Medical Residency Certification Board® (AMRCB®)

Association of American Medical Colleges

Association of Faculties of Medicine of Canada (AFMC)

Association of International Physicians and Surgeons of Nova Scotia

Best 167 Medical Schools, 2015 Edition. The Princeton Review

Canadian Federation of Medical Students

Canadian Medical Association

Canadian Medical Association Masterfile, 2014

Canadian Medical Education Statistics publication - http://www.afmc.ca/publications-statistics-e.php

Canadian Policy Research Networks (CPRN)

Canadian Post-M.D. Education Registry (CAPER)

Canadian Resident Matching Services

Canadian Students Studying Medicine Abroad, Canadian Resident Matching Service. Copyright October 2010.

College of Family Physicians of Canada

College of Physicians and Surgeons of Ontario (CPSO)

Committee on Accreditation of Canadian Medical Schools (CACMS)

Committee on Accreditation of Continuing Medical Education (CACME)

Council on Medical Education and Hospitals, American Medical Association, 1918

Department of Human Resources and Social Development Canada

Foundation for Advancement of International Medical Education and Research (FAIMER)

Framework for Collaborative Pan-Canadian Health Human Resources Planning

KW Eva, J Rosenfeld, HI Reiter and GR Norman (2004a). An admissions OSCE: the multiple mini-interview. Medical Education 38:314-326.

KW Eva, J Rosenfeld, HI Reiter and GR Norman (2004b). The ability of the multiple mini-interview to predict pre-clerkship performance in medical school. Academic Medicine 79:S40-S42.

KW Eva, J Rosenfeld, HI Reiter and GR Norman (2004c). The relationship between interviewers' characteristics and ratings assigned during a multiple mini-interview. Academic Medicine 79:602-609.

HW Reiter and KW Eva (2005). Reflecting the relative values of community, faculty, and students in the admissions tools of medical schools. Teach Learn Med 17(1)L 4-8.

J Rosenfeld, HI Reiter and GR Norman (2004c). The relationship between interviewers' characteristics and ratings assigned during a multiple mini-interview. Academic Medicine 79:602-609.

International Medical Education Directory (IMED)

Liaison Committee on Medical Education (LCME)

Medical School Admission Requirements (MSAR®), 2012-2013. Association of American Medical Colleges

National Assessment Collaboration (NAC)

National Matching Services Inc. (NMS)

Office of Research and Information Services (ORIS). The Associations of Faculties of Medicine of Canada

Ontario Medical School Application Service (OMSAS)

Society for Canadians Studying Medicine Abroad

Royal College of Physicians and Surgeons of Canada (RCPSC)

Thomson and Cohl, 2011 – Ontario Medical Report.

World Medical Association

http://en.wikipedia.org/wiki/List_of_medical_schools_in_Canada

http://en.wikipedia.org/wiki/Medical_Council_of_Canada

http://en.wikipedia.org/wiki/Medical_school_in_Canada

http://en.wikipedia.org/wiki/Student_loans_in_Canada

http://mcc.ca/home/

http://mcc.ca/examinations/nac-overview/

http://mcc.ca/examinations/self-administered-exam/

http://www.afmc.ca/pdf/datapoint/IMG-CSA_DataPoint_update_Jan-2014.pdf

http://www.afmc.ca/pdf/DataPoint_Oct_2010_eng.pdf

http://www.afmc.ca/pdf/datapoint/DATAPOINT-may-eng.pdf

http://www.afmc.ca/pdf/DataPoint_Sept_2008_eng.pdf

http://www.carms.ca/en/match-process/match-timelines/

http://www.carms.ca/assets/upload/pdfs/2010_CSA_Report/CaRMS_2010_CSA_Report.pdf

http://www.cfpc.ca/FMExam/

https://www.cibc.com/ca/loans/articles/student-loan-guide.html

http://www.faimer.org/resources/imed.html

http://www.ivyglobal.ca/MCAT/med_schools_canada.asp

http://www.mcgill.ca/medcareerplan/2-exploring-options/usmle

http://www.ncbi.nlm.nih.gov/pmc/articles/PMC3374698/

http://www.womenscollegehospital.ca/about-us/our-history/

CONTACT ORGANIZATIONS

American Association of Colleges of Osteopathic Medicine (AACOM)
550 Friendship Boulevard
Suite 310
Chevy Chase, MD 20815-7231
Tel: 301-968-4100
Fax: 301-968-4101

American Association of Medical Colleges (AAMC)
2450 N. Street, Northwest
Washington, DC 20037-1126
Tel: 202-828-0400
Fax: 202-828-1125
www.aamc.org

American Medical Residency Certification Board® (AMRCB®)
The Prudential Tower
800 Boylston Street, 16th Floor
Boston, MA 02199
www.amrcb.com

American Osteopathic Organization (AOA)
142 East Ontario Street
Chicago, IL 60611-2864
Tel: 802-621-1773
Fax: 312-202-8200
www.osteopathic.org

The Association of Faculties of Medicine of Canada (AFMC)
265 Carling Avenue, Suite 800
Ottawa, Ontario, Canada K1S 2E1
Phone: 613-730-0687, ext. 225 or 270
Fax: 613-730-1196
Email: cacms@afmc.ca

Educational Commission for Foreign Medical Graduates (ECFMG)
3624 Market Street
Philadelphia, PA 19104-2685
Tel: 265-386-5900
Fax: 215-386-9196
www.ecfmg.org

Federation of State Medical Boards
PO Box 619850
Dallas, TX 75261-9850
Tel: 817-868-4000
Fax: 817-868-4099
www.fsmb.org

National Board of Medical Examiners
3750 Market Street
Philadelphia, PA 19104-3102
Tel: 215-590-9500
Fax: 215-590-9457
www.nbme.org

Ontario Medical School Application Service (OMSAS)
Ontario Universities' Application Centre
170 Research Lane
Guelph ON N1G 5E2
Tel.: 519-823-1940
Fax: 519-823-5232
E-mail: omsas@ouac.on.ca
Web-site: www.ouac.on.ca/omsas

STUDENT DISCOUNTS AND ADVERTISING

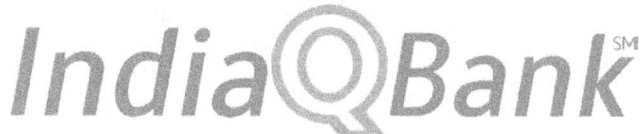

Prepare with Confidence!

Are you looking for quality, expert and accurate prep questions created by expert physicians? The American Medical Residency Certification Board® (AMRCB®) has partnered with IndiaQBank to offer an online study tool at a **25%** discount! IndiaQBank is an online study tool for helping you study and pass your AIPGMEE, FMGE, USMLE or JEE Mains boards.

If you identify an affiliation with the AMRCB® you will receive **25% off** the subscription that best fits your needs.

1. Access IndiaQBank question banks at www.indiaqbank.com
2. Sign-up by entering your name and email, choose a password and agree to terms and conditions.
3. Choose the test bank and the subscription that best fits your needs. IndiaQBank has multiple subscription terms to choose from.
4. When checking out, enter the code AMRCB for a **25%** discount off the purchase price.

- IndiaQBank is an online test preparation service for the Medical and Engineering exams of India.
- IndiaQBank features accuracy and expertise in question and case creation that will give you the very best studying preparation experience available for you to pass your Medical or Engineering Exam.
- Our MCQs and explanations have been created by expert physicians and engineers.
- The questions encountered on the qbank have been shown to mirror the exact questions encountered on the actual licensing exams.

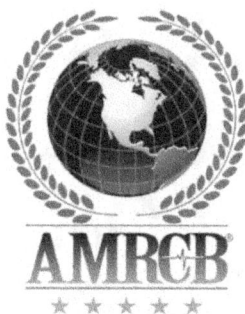

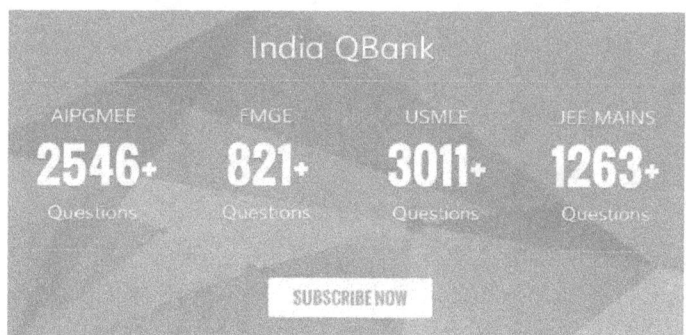

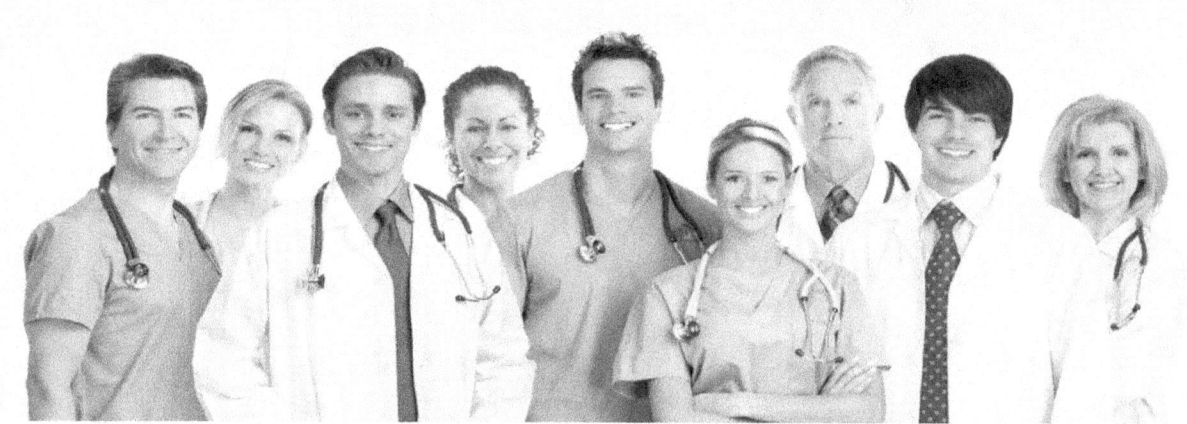

Enhance Physician Training Via the #1 Source for Specialty Medical Education

WHAT IS BOARDVITALS?

BoardVitals™ is the largest and most used question bank for In-Service exams, Board Exams, Shelf Exams, and Physician Re-Certifications. We provide 20,000 questions, answers, and explanations targeted to over 20 medical and other healthcare specialities

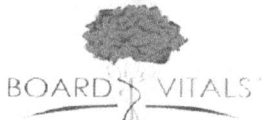

BoardVitals TestBanks
Cardiology Child
Psychiatry
Dermatology Echo
Emergency Medicine ENT
Family Medicine GI
Internal Medicine
Neurology OBGYN
Pathology
Pediatrics
Psychiatry
Psychiatry Vignettes
Radiology
Surgery Shelf
Exams
USMLE Step 1
USMLE Step 2
USMLE Step 3

If you identify an affiliation with AMRCB using the links and steps below, you can purchase BoardVitals products at **10% off the individual price.**

1. Access BoardVitals products at:
   http://vwww.boardvitals.com/

2. Choose the test bank and the subscription term that best fits your needs: 1 Month, 3 Months or 6 Months

3. Enter your name and e-mail, choose a password and agree to the terms and conditions.

4. When checking out, enter in the code AMRCB for a 10% discount off the purchase price.

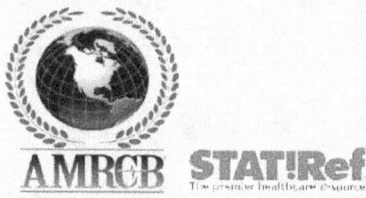

PCS
Practitioner Contracting Services

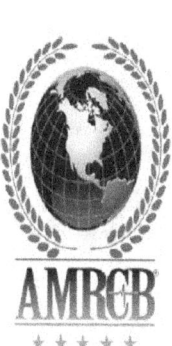

AMRCB is excited to partner with Practitioner Contracting Services to offer our clients an expert team to assist them in career planning. PCS offers over 30 years of combined experience in Health Law and now offers contract negotiations and career planning services to medical students, medical school, residents, fellows and practicing physicians. As a corporate partner with AMRCB, PCS offers a 20% discount to all AMRCB clients. The PCS fee is a flat fee, instead of the hourly fee you will find at most locations and companies. You can rest assured that no matter what comes your way, or how long it takes, your fee has been paid and it will cover everything.

For Medical Students: For our medical students PCS offers both Personal Statement review and Visa guidance. Personal statements are the first thing potential residency programs see; along with your CV and test scores. It is vital that students make a great first impression with their personal statements and are able to convey all the wonderful attributes they bring to the table. PCS can assist with personal statements in all stages of completion; from helping you get started, helping you draft a statement, knowing what to include, grammar and typographical editing and creative writing review and assistance.

In addition to personal statement review, PCS offers Visa guidance. For many international students the Visa process can be very complicated and confusing; but PCS helps to eliminate those concerns. PCS assists student as they maneuver what forms need to be filed with which governmental agencies, how the process will work and what to expect along the way.

For Residents and Fellows: For residents, fellows and practicing physicians PCS offers both Visa guidance and contract review and negotiation. Along with the Visa guidance services discussed above, PCS also can assist physicians as they receive employment contracts with their chosen practice. PCS will review each contract to ensure it offers the best salary, benefits, avoids pitfalls and problem terms and offers the best protection for the physician. From start to finish, all aspects of the negotiation is included in the PCS service fee.

www.Practitionercontractingservices.com or call 1-904-342-7390

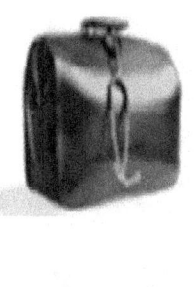

ATTENDINGDR

What is AttendingDr?

AttendingDr is a professional HIPAA-secure networking platform centered around the needs of physicians, built by practicing physicians. Whether you're a doctor or administrator in private practice or a hospital, AttendingDr serves to provide invaluable resources for your work and career. The platform includes a robust HIPAA-secure messaging, state-of-the-art patient referral system and scheduling software, Telemedicine platform, physicians' career center, credentialing system, and access to member benefits. Current member benefits include HIPAA-Insurance, discounts for malpractice, disability, and other insurance products, access to marketing assistance, and many other benefits. All this in a secure environment that will ensure privacy and security of your information.

AttendingDr was created with the collaboration of ideas from physicians, healthcare industry executives, and entrepreneurs. Join today or Inquire about our private white label solutions for your organization.

Visit **www.attendingdr.com** today!

www.ingramcontent.com/pod-product-compliance
Lightning Source LLC
Chambersburg PA
CBHW080806180526
45168CB00006B/2346

* 9 7 8 1 5 0 7 8 1 7 1 7 9 *